Key Clinical Trials in
Erectile Dysfunction

Culley C. Carson

Key Clinical Trials in Erectile Dysfunction

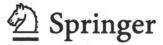 Springer

Culley C. Carson, MD, FACS
Rhodes Distinguished Professor
Chief of Urology
Division of Urologic Surgery
University of North Carolina at Chapel Hill
Chapel Hill, NC, USA

British Library Cataloguing in Publication Data
A catalogue record for this book is available from the British Library

Library of Congress Control Number: 2006923813

ISBN-10: 1-84628-427-9   e-ISBN-10: 1-84628-428-7
ISBN-13: 978-1-84628-427-4   e-ISBN-13: 978-1-84628-428-1

Printed on acid-free paper

9 8 7 6 5 4 3 2 1

Springer Science+Business Media, LLC

Contents

Abbreviations

AE	Adverse Event
BP	Blood Pressure
BSFI	Brief Sexual Function Index
CR	Controlled Release
CUMRI	Cavernosal Unstriated Muscle Relaxant Injection
ED	Erectile Dysfunction
FSH	Follicle Stimulating Hormone
i.c.	intracavernous
IIEF	International Index for Erectile Dysfunction
MUSE	Medicated Urethral System for Erection
NPTR	Nocturnal Penile Tumescence Rigidity
PGE_1	Prostaglandin E_1
RN	Rigiscan Number
RTM	Real Time Monitoring
SCI	Spinal Cord Injury
SL	Sublingual
VAS	Visual Analogue Scale
VSS	Visual Sexual Stimulation

1. Study Descriptor

The Earliest Carefully Controlled Clinical Trial Evaluating Oral Pharmacotherapy (Yohimbine) in ED

1.1 KEY TRIAL REFERENCES

1.1.1 Major Publication
Miller W. Afrodex in the treatment of male impotence: a double-blind crossover study. Curr Ther Res 10(7):354–359, 1968.

1.1.2 Other Important Publications
Margolis R, Prieto P, et al. Statistical analysis of 10,000 male cases using Afrodex in treatment of impotence. Curr Ther Res Exp 13(9): 616–622, 1971.

Roberts C, Sloboda W. Afrodex vs. placebo in the treatment of male impotence: statistical analysis of two double-blind crossover studies. Curr Ther Res Clin Exp 16(1):96–99, 1974.

1.2 IMPORTANCE OF STUDY
This was one of the first carefully controlled studies of erectile dysfunction that used a placebo. It is also important insofar as it was the first rigorous analysis of the claimed erectogenic properties of yohimbine.

1.3 STUDY DESIGN
Double-blind, placebo-controlled, crossover study. n = 22.

The patients were divided into 2 groups. Group A (n = 12) received Regimen A (Afrodex – Nux vomica extract 5 mg, methyl testosterone 5 mg, and yohimbine 5 mg) t.i.d. for 4 weeks, followed by a 2-week washout and then regimen B (placebo) t.i.d. for a further 4 weeks. For group B (n = 10), regimens A and B were reversed.

1.3.1 Outcome Measures
Number of erections and number of orgasms attained in the previous week. Patients were evaluated at 2-week intervals for the duration of the study.

1.3.2 Inclusion Criteria
Men with impotence (age range, 29–62 years; duration of impotence, 2 weeks – 5 years).

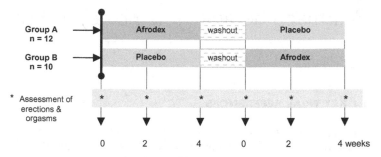

FIGURE 1.1. Yohimbine (Afrodex) study randomization scheme

1.4 KEY RESULTS
- For Group A (Afrodex first), potency improved during the 4-week Afrodex therapy by 222% and 300% in the number of erections and orgasms, respectively, and there was no significant loss of potency during the 2-week washout period (–14% and –6% for erections and orgasms, respectively). With placebo therapy, this group experienced a 40% increase in erections and a 17% increase in orgasms.
- For Group B (placebo first), potency improved during the 4-week placebo therapy by 566% and 433% in the number of erections and orgasms, respectively, but there was a more significant loss of potency during the 2-week washout period (–30% and –50% for erections and orgasms, respectively). With Afrodex therapy, the group then experienced a 118% increase in erections and a 300% increase in orgasms.
- Combined data for both groups show that Afrodex therapy resulted in increases in the number of erections and orgasms of 165% and 300%, respectively. Similarly, placebo therapy resulted in increases of 96% and 55%.
- No significant side effects were noted.

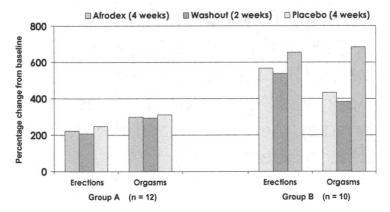

FIGURE 1.2. Efficacy of Afrodex compared with placebo for the treatment of impotence (determined by number of erections and orgasms per week)

1.5 CONCLUSIONS FROM ORIGINAL REPORTS
In this double-blind, crossover study, a substantial placebo effect did not demonstrate the importance of psychological factors in the syndrome of impotence.

However, the results also indicate that Afrodex is 1.7 times more effective than placebo in relieving impotence, as measured by increase in the number of erections. Similarly, Afrodex was 5.4 times more effective, as measured by the number of orgasms.

1.6 STRENGTHS
The trial design would be considered "gold standard" 30 years later in many ways. In particular, a crossover design in which each patient was exposed to active drug and placebo was incorporated.

1.7 WEAKNESSES
The lack of a questionnaire, such as the International Index for Erectile Dysfunction (IIEF) in the 1990s is an obvious disadvantage, although the basic conclusions are valid. Because the product also contained a small dose of methyl testosterone, it is not possible to unequivocally assign any benefit to yohimbine alone.

1.8 RELEVANCE
The conclusions of this study have stood the test of time, in that yohimbine monotherapy has only a modest beneficial effect in ED patients.

The relatively modest effects accounted for the considerable lack of interest in pharmacotherapy prior to early intracavernosal studies.

2. Study Descriptor

A Description of the Pioneering
Work That Led to the First
Approved Agents for ED: Giles
Brindley, the Needle, and the Penis
(Phenoxybenzamine)

2.1 KEY TRIAL REFERENCES

2.1.1 Major Publication

Brindley G. Cavernosal alpha-blockade: a new technique for investigating and treating erectile dysfunction. Br J Psychiat 143:332–337, 1983.

2.1.2 Other Important Publications

Virag R. Intracavernous injection of papaverine for erectile failure. Lancet ii, 938, 1982.

Brindley G. Maintenance treatment of erectile impotence by cavernosal unstriated muscle relaxant injection. Br J Psychiat 149:210–215, 1986.

Keogh E, Earle C, et al. Treatment of impotence by intrapenile injections of papaverine and phenoxybenzamine: a double-blind controlled trial. Aust NZ J Med 19(2):108–112, 1989.

2.2 IMPORTANCE OF STUDY

Although some earlier work had been described by Virag, this study really laid down the foundation for the use of therapeutics in the management of ED. It encouraged both patients and physicians to believe that there was a realistic alternative to corrective or implant surgery.

2.3 STUDY DESIGN

Prospective Trial. n = 15.

The results of 47 cavernosal α-blockade injections in 15 subjects are reported. Phenoxybenzamine was used at dosages of 2.5 to 7 mg in 10 ml saline.

2.3.1 Outcome Measures

Presence and duration of erection, latency to tumescence, quality of erection (not doublable, not flexible to right angle, fully erect), and occurrence of ejaculation/coitus were recorded, as well as systemic and local adverse events (AEs).

2.3.2 Inclusion Criteria

Potent (n = 4) and impotent (n = 11) men. Subjects were initially assessed for the presence of erections during masturbation and on waking. The age range of the patients was 20 to 64 years, and the duration of impotence ranged from 11 months to 22 years. The 4 potent men were all healthy, but 2 were anorgasmic. Of the impotent men, 5 were healthy, 1 was diabetic, 1 was schizophrenic, 3 had spinal injuries, and 1 had multiple sclerosis.

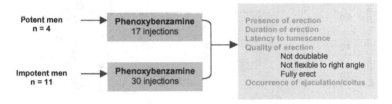

FIGURE 2.1. Phenoxybenzamine injecton trial study design

2.4 KEY RESULTS

- Of 17 injections performed in the 4 potent men (2 of whom were anorgasmic), 10 resulted in full erections, ranging in duration from 1 to 4 hours. Partial erections (penis not "doublable") were achieved in 16 of the 17 injections, ranging from 1–5 hours.

- Of 30 injections performed in the 11 impotent men, 17 resulted in full erections, ranging in duration from 1–30 hours. Partial erections resulted from 29 of these injections, ranging from 1–30 hours. There was some degree of erectile response from every injection in this group.

- Prolonged full erections occurred in 2 subjects. The first man was had a full erection for 30 hours after 3 of 6 injections but was not distressed and engaged in coitus twice on each occasion. The other man had a full erection for 6 hours on 2 occasions and a prolonged and painful erection for 22 hours on a third occasion, which required intervention.

- The erections induced by phenoxybenzamine enabled 6 of the impotent men to have sexual intercourse.
- Transient pain was experienced in and around the glans of the penis (distal from the injection site) with these injections, usually nonsevere and lasting 2 to 5 minutes.
- Only 2 systemic adverse events (AEs) were noted with this technique; one man noticed sweating on his trunk during and for a few minutes after his first injection, and another had dry orgasms after 2 of 11 injections.

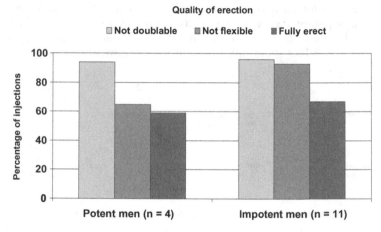

FIGURE 2.2. Induction of penile erection by intracavernosal injection of phenoxybenzamine in potent and impotent men

2.5 CONCLUSIONS FROM ORIGINAL REPORTS

Intracavernosal injection of phenoxybenzamine (2.5–7 mg) was effective in producing erections in potent and impotent men.

The duration of erection (<30 hours) produced by this technique is unpredictable, with the risk of prolonged and painful erections. Further understanding of the physiological mechanisms involved in this technique should improve predictability.

2.6 STRENGTHS

The real strength of the study was that, in the absence of any real information, patients were prepared to volunteer.

2.7 WEAKNESSES

The study did not include a placebo and was performed on only 11 patients. However, many subsequent studies have shown the placebo effect to be negligible.

2.8 RELEVANCE

Although phenoxybenzamine has largely been replaced by prostaglandin E_1 (PGE_1) and mixes of vasorelaxant agents, until the arrival of sildenafil intracavernosal administration was the mainstay of therapy. Even after the arrival of sildenafil, there is still relatively widespread use of injectables, and indeed some patients prefer the quality of the erection achieved.

3. Study Descriptor

The Pivotal Study Showing That Intracorporal Injection of Vasoactive Agents (Papaverine or Phenoxybenzamine) Was Effective Pharmacotherapy

3.1 KEY TRIAL REFERENCES

3.1.1 Major Publication
Brindley G. Maintenance treatment of erectile impotence by cavernosal unstriated muscle relaxant injection. Br J Psychiat 149:210–215, 1986.

3.1.2 Other Important Publications
Brindley S. Pilot experiments on the actions of drugs injected into the human corpus cavernosum penis. Br J Pharmacol 87(3):495–500, 1986.

Szasz G, Stevenson R, et al. Induction of penile erection by intracavernosal injection: a double-blind comparison of phenoxybenzamine versus papaverine-phentolamine versus saline. Arch Sex Behav 16(5):371–379, 1987.

3.2 IMPORTANCE OF STUDY
Although intracavernosal administration had been performed several years before, the work described here provided important additional information to the physician insofar as the erectile response could be achieved with any vasorelaxant agent, not just phenoxybenzamine.

3.3 STUDY DESIGN
Prospective, long-term study. n = 127.

This study reports on the use of Cavernosal Unstriated Muscle Relaxant Injection (CUMRI) using papaverine (16–40 mg) or phenoxybenzamine (4–10 mg) for the investigation and treatment of erectile impotence.

Initially, injections of papaverine were used, the duration of erectile response was assessed, and if it was insufficient, phenoxybenzamine was used.

For 73 patients, the selected agent was self-administered at home.

3.3.1 Outcome Measures

Erection sufficient for coitus, treatment success or failure (defined as continued use of CUMRI at home).

3.3.2 Inclusion Criteria

Men with erectile impotence of various etiologies. Forty-six patients had spinal cord injuries or disease (36 patients with spinal cord injury, 7 with multiple sclerosis, 1 with poliomyelitis, and 1 paraplegic), and 81 other patients most of whom had no known relevant disease. Age range, 20 to 79 years.

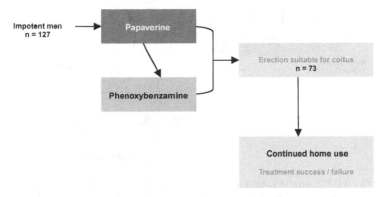

FIGURE 3.1. Papaverine to phentolamine crossover study design and randomization

3.4 KEY RESULTS

- In 113 of 127 patients CUMRI with papaverine or phenoxybenzamine (n = 26) resulted in erections suitable for coitus (i.e., stiff enough to resist bending in the middle of the shaft by 45°), for 20 continuous minutes.
- In the remaining 14 patients, this degree of erection was not achieved, although a larger dose might have been successful. Failure was significantly more common in older patients.

- Of the 113 patients with a positive erectile response, 73 used the technique at home. At the end of the study, 54 patients were still using CUMRI at home and 19 had used it but no longer did so. Reasons for discontinuation of CUMRI included symptom improvement (3), loss of efficacy (2), loss of sexual partner (2), implantation of penile prosthesis (1), and death (1 from unrelated myocardial infarction).
- Most patients experienced mild burning pain after injection of either agent, lasting 10 to 15 minutes with phenoxybenzamine and <2 minutes with papaverine.
- Priapism (continuous erection ≥12 hours) occurred in 11 patients (16 injections); 4 resolved spontaneously and 12 required intervention. The cause was phenoxybenzamine in 4 cases and papaverine in 12.

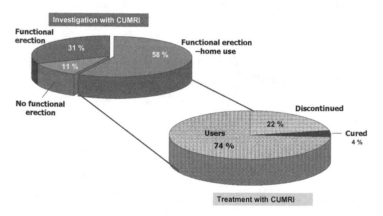

FIGURE 3.2. Investigation and treatment of erectile impotence by cavernosal unstriated muscle relaxant injection (CUMRI) using papaverine or phenoxybenzamine

3.5 CONCLUSIONS FROM ORIGINAL REPORTS

The technique of CUMRI using papaverine or phenoxybenzamine was effective in causing erections sufficient for coitus in the majority (89%) of impotent patients. Of the patients who used CUMRI at home, 74% continued to use it and were satisfied with the treatment.

CUMRI as a diagnostic technique is useful in confirming the integrity of the arterial supply outside the penis (internal iliac arteries and relevant branches), which is required to support a full erection. The success of CUMRI will probably exclude cavernoso-venous or cavernoso-spongiosal shunts as the sole or principal cause of impotence.

3.6 STRENGTHS
In this study Brindley circumvented the major limitation of his earlier study by using over 100 patients. The overall response rate convinced many urologists that intracorporal administration was a viable option.

3.7 WEAKNESSES
There was no placebo group in the study, and the assessment of efficacy was somewhat subjective.

3.8 RELEVANCE
This study has stood the test of time. For almost a decade, intracavernosal administration was widely used. Although they have been replaced to a large extent by oral agents, there is still considerable use of injectables.

4. Study Descriptor

The First Placebo-Controlled Study on the Benefits of Intracorporal Administration of Vasorelaxant Agents to ED Patients (Papaverine/Phentolamine Combination)

4.1 KEY TRIAL REFERENCES

4.1.1 Major Publication

Kiely E, Ignotus P, and Williams G. Penile function following intracavernosal injection of vasoactive agents or saline. Br J Urol 59:473–476, 1987.

4.1.2 Other Important Publications

Williams G, Mulcahy M, and Kiely E. Impotence: treatment by auto-injection of vasoactive drugs. Br Med J (Clin Res Ed) 5;295(6598): 596–596, 1987.

Kiely E, Bloom S, and Williams G. Penile response to intracavernosal vasoactive intestinal polypeptide alone and in combination with other vasoactive agents. Br J Urol 64(2):191–194, 1989.

Armstrong D, Convery A, and Dinsmore W. Intracavernosal papaverine and phentolamine for the medical management of erectile dysfunction in a genitourinary clinic. Int J STD AIDS 4(4):214–216, 1993.

Dinsmore W, Alderdice D. Vasoactive intestinal polypeptide and phentolamine mesylate administered by autoinjection in the treatment of patients with erectile dysfunction resistant to other intracavernosal agents. Br J Urol 81(3):437–440, 1998.

4.2 IMPORTANCE OF STUDY

Although somewhat limited by patient numbers, this study unequivocally demonstrated that there is a negligible placebo response and that there is considerable clinical benefit from the injection of vasoactive agents.

4.3 STUDY DESIGN

Double-blind, crossover study. n = 18.

Patients were randomized to receive a single injection of either 2 ml of saline or 2 ml of solution containing papaverine (30 mg) and phentolamine (1 mg). The immediate response to the injection and also any change in erectile function over the subsequent 4 weeks were documented. The procedure was then repeated with patients crossing over to the other regimen.

4.3.1 Outcome Measures

Immediate erectile response. Recording change in penile length and rigidity (visual and tactile assessment) and rating using the Penrig scale.

Penrig scale:		
	<10	no change in size of penis
	10–30	change in volume and size, no rigidity
	30–50	tumescence present
	50–75	tumescence is clear, erection starts
	75–80	rigidity achieved
	>100	completely rigid

Subsequent spontaneous erections. During 4-week follow-up, spontaneous erections were graded as A (none), B (improvement, better erection but insufficient for intercourse), or C (normal intercourse possible when attempted).

4.3.2 Inclusion Criteria

Impotent men (psychogenic 7, organic 11). The age range was 22 to 65 years.

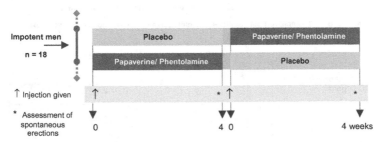

FIGURE 4.1. Papaverine/phentolamine versus placebo study of impotent men: crossover design

4.4 KEY RESULTS

- Among those patients who received saline as their first injection (n = 8), there was no immediate erectile response in any patient, and only 1 patient experienced an improvement in spontaneous erections during the subsequent 4 weeks (grade B for 3 weeks).
- However, in this same group, all patients experienced an immediate erectile response with the phentolamine/papaverine injection (mean Penrig score, 72.5). Four of these patients were subsequently able to have sexual intercourse (grade C for 1–3 weeks), and improvement in spontaneous erections was reported in 2 patients (grade B for 3 weeks).
- In the group that received phentolamine/papaverine as the first injection (n = 10), all patients had an immediate response (mean Penrig score, 67.5). Three of these patients were able to have intercourse for the 4 weeks following and 4 other patients for the first week. The remaining 3 patients showed no improvement in spontaneous erections.
- For these 10 patients, there was no immediate erectile response with saline. During the following 4 weeks, 4 of 7 patients who had achieved normal erections with phentolamine/papaverine continued to have spontaneous erections but insufficient for intercourse (grade B), 2 reverted to having no erections (grade A), and only 1 patient continued to have functional erections. The 3 patients who had not responded to phentolamine/papaverine also did not respond to saline.
- No adverse events were reported with either injection.

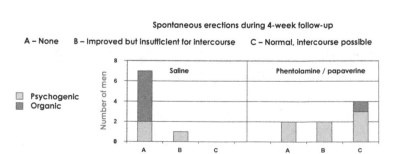

FIGURE 4.2. Penile function following a single intracavernosal injection of phentolamine/papaverine of saline in impotent men

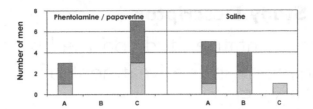

FIGURE 4.2. *Continued*

4.5 CONCLUSIONS FROM ORIGINAL REPORTS

This study shows the effectiveness of intracavernosal injections of vasoactive agents (phentolamine and papaverine) in treating impotence of various etiologies (psychogenic, neuropathic, and arteriogenic).

All patients showed an immediate response to phentolamine/papaverine injection and, 72% of patients reported improvements in their spontaneous erections during the subsequent 1 to 4 weeks.

These results also suggest that any placebo effect is minimal in this group of patients, in which there is a considerable psychogenic overlay to their impotence.

4.6 STRENGTHS

The major advantage of this small study was that it showed that there was no placebo response to intracavernosal injection. The study design was an elegant crossover one.

4.7 WEAKNESSES

The somewhat limited number of patients would nowadays be considered a disadvantage.

4.8 RELEVANCE

From this trial onwards, it was possible to conclude that there was next to no placebo response to injections into the corpus cavernosum. Several of the men in this study had also been exposed to papaverine alone, with a somewhat more limited response. On this basis, it could be argued that this trial laid down the foundation for the successful subsequent use of combinations of vasoactive agents.

5. Study Descriptor

Representative Study on the Use of Yohimbine in the Treatment of Organic ED

5.1 KEY TRIAL REFERENCES

5.1.1 Major Publication
Morales A, Condra M, et al. Is yohimbine effective in the control of organic impotence? Results of a controlled trial. J Urol 237:1168–1172, 1987.

5.1.2 Other Important Publications
Reid K, Surridge D, et al. Double-blind trial of yohimbine in treatment of psychogenic impotence. Lancet 22;2(8556):421–423, 1987.

Susset J, Tessier C, et al. Effect of yohimbine hydrochloride on erectile impotence: a double-blind study. J Urol 141(6):1360–1363, 1989.

Vogt H, Brandl P, et al. Double-blind, placebo-controlled safety and efficacy trial with yohimbine hydrochloride in the treatment of non-organic erectile dysfunction. Int J Impot Res 9(3):155–161, 1997.

Morales A. Yohimbine in erectile dysfunction: the facts. Int J Impot Res 12 (Suppl 1): S70–74, 2000.

5.2 IMPORTANCE OF STUDY
Although by no means the first study on the use of yohimbine in the treatment of ED, in many respects this is the defining one. In this adequately powered, placebo-controlled study, yohimbine monotherapy was shown to have only a modest effect beyond that of placebo.

5.3 STUDY DESIGN
Randomized, double-blind, placebo-controlled, partial crossover study. n = 100.

Men were randomized to receive orally either yohimbine (6 mg with riboflavin marker) or placebo (riboflavin), three times daily for 10 weeks. Riboflavin was used to check patient compliance to medication (urinary riboflavin being easily detected by fluorescence). At the end of this treatment phase, the blind was broken. Those patients who had received placebo during phase

1 were given yohimbine, and those who had taken yohimbine were permitted to continue if their response to the drug had been positive. Patients were then treated for a further 10 weeks.

5.3.1 Outcome Measures

Patient and partner interviews were conducted at the end of each treatment phase (10 weeks) to determine therapeutic response. Response to treatment was classified as:

Complete response. Patient reported complete return to satisfactory sexual functioning with erections sufficient for penetration (confirmed by partner).
Partial response. Patient and partner reported some improvement in quality of erections (frequency or rigidity) but insufficient to restore satisfactory sexual performance.
Failure. Patient and partner reported no change in erectile functioning from pretreatment levels.

Compliance with medication was checked at weeks 4, 7, and 10 during each phase.

5.3.2 Inclusion Criteria

Men aged 18 to 70 years with impotence of a definite organic etiology and continuous failure for ≥3 months to attain erection sufficient for intromission.

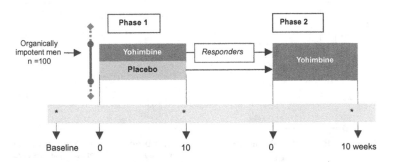

FIGURE 5.1. Yohimbine versus placebo in impotent men: crossover design

5.4 KEY RESULTS

- Of the patients who received yohimbine in phase 1, 42.6% reported a positive response (21.3% complete, 21.3% partial response).
- Of the patients who received placebo during phase 1, 27.6% reported a positive response (13.8% complete, 13.8% partial response).
- Although the data for yohimbine were favorable, they did not reach statistical significance (p = 0.42).
- At the end of phase 2, 45.5% of the patients who had taken placebo during phase 1 reported a positive response (18.2% complete, 27.3% partial response) to yohimbine.
- The combined (phases 1 and 2) response rates to yohimbine were positive for 43.5% (20.3% complete, 23.2% partial response).
- A further analysis was performed to ascertain the characteristics of the responders (age, penile brachial index, testosterone, follicle stimulating hormone [FSH], prolactin, diabetic status, presence of paresthesia, presence of peripheral vascular disease, and concomitant antihypertensive medications). No consistent differences emerged between responders and nonresponders.

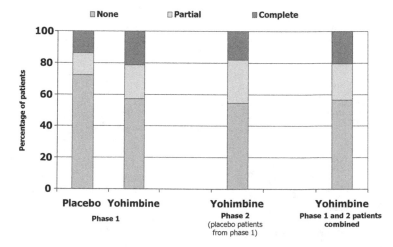

FIGURE 5.2. Treatment response to yohimbine in organically impotent men (determined by self-report after 10 weeks of therapy)

5.5 CONCLUSIONS FROM ORIGINAL REPORTS

The response rate to oral yohimbine in organically impotent men is marginal.

Adrenoreceptors are involved in the erectile process, but other neurotransmitter systems also are putative modulators (cholinergic, dopaminergic, vasoactive intestinal polypeptide), and thus it could not be expected that a single agent would be useful in all cases of organic impotence.

However, because of its ease of administration and safety, yohimbine is a treatment option for those patients who do not accept more invasive methods.

5.6 STRENGTHS

The patient population and inclusion criteria were rigorously defined at baseline. An attempt was also made to stratify the comorbidities in the ED patients to determine if these could influence the interpretation. The group size (100) was large.

5.7 WEAKNESSES

As would be expected for a study from this era, the endpoints used in the evaluation were somewhat subjective and were not necessarily consistent throughout the course of the study.

5.8 RELEVANCE

This study is entirely predictive of the wider-scale clinical evaluation and use of yohimbine. In a general patient population, the drug has only minimal effect when administered as monotherapy, although the effect may be greater in psychogenic ED. However, the use of yohimbine as part of a drug combination cannot be discounted.

6. Study Descriptor

Defining the Therapeutic Ratio for Intracavernosal Administration of Prostaglandin E_1 (Alprostadil)

6.1 KEY TRIAL REFERENCES

6.1.1 Major Publication
Linet O, Ogrinc F. Efficacy and safety of intracavernosal alprostadil in men with erectile dysfunction. N Engl J Med 334:873–877, 1996.

6.1.2 Other Important Publications
Linet O, Neff L. Intracavernous prostaglandin E_1 in erectile dysfunction. Clin Invest 72:139–149, 1989.

Brock G, Tu L, Linet O. Return of spontaneous erection during long-term intracavernosal alprostadil (Caverject) treatment. Urology 57(3): 536–541, 2001.

6.2 STUDY FUNDING
Upjohn Company

6.3 IMPORTANCE OF STUDY
Although intracavernosal administration of prostaglandin E_1 (PGE_1) had been performed since the mid-1980s, few data were available from reliable clinical trials. This study provided a rigorous clinical rationale for the continued use of intracorporal PGE_1.

6.4 STUDY DESIGN
Three multicenter, prospective trials. n = 296, 201, and 683.

Dose-response study. In this parallel, double-blind, placebo-controlled study, 296 men were randomized to receive a single 1-ml intracavernosal injection of placebo (n = 59) or alprostadil in doses of 2.5 µg (n = 57), 5 µg (n = 60), 10 µg (n = 62), or 20 µg (n = 58).

Dose-finding study. In this single-blind study, 201 men received increasing doses of intracavernosal alprostadil (0.5, 1, 2, 3, 4,

5, 7.5, 10, 15, 20, 25, and 30μg) at intervals of 2 to 14 days, until a minimal effective dose was established (>70% rigidity lasting >10 minutes by Rigiscan testing) or the maximum dose was reached.

Efficacy and safety study. An open-label, flexible-dose study in 683 men with stable sexual relationships. The optimal dose of alprostadil was established for each man (erection sufficient for vaginal penetration and lasting ≤60 minutes) by dose titration. Patients then used self-injection therapy at home and were followed for 6 months.

6.4.1 Outcome Measures

Dose-response and dose-finding studies. Penile rigidity was determined by palpation (absent, partial, or full [sufficient for intercourse]) at specified times after injection. Rigidity was also measured by Rigiscan prior to injection and for 2 hours after, a response being >70% rigidity at base or tip lasting >10 consecutive minutes. Duration of erection was also measured.

Efficacy and safety study. Patient diaries recorded; frequency of drug use, evaluations of erections (none, partial, full), and evaluations of intercourse (satisfactory or unsatisfactory). Partners were also asked to rate satisfaction of intercourse. Adverse events were reported by diaries and enquiry.

6.4.2 Inclusion Criteria

Men with erectile dysfunction (vasculogenic, neurogenic, psychogenic, or mixed origin) lasting at least 4 months.

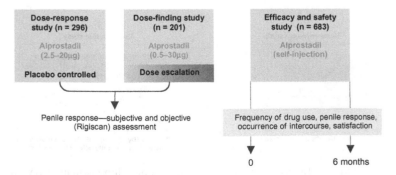

FIGURE 6.1. Alprostadil intracavernosal injection study: study design

6.5 KEY RESULTS

- *Dose-response study.* All doses of alprostadil were superior to placebo, and there was a significant dose–response relationship with increasing doses of alprostadil (from 2.5 to 20 µg) for both clinical and Rigiscan evaluations. The mean duration of erection ranged from 12 minutes after the 2.5-µg dose to 44 minutes after the 20-µg dose. Penile pain was reported by 23% of men who received alprostadil, but was not dose related.

- *Dose-finding study.* One hundred thirty-five men (67%) completed the study. The minimal effective dose was ≤2 µg in 38%, 23%, 20%, and 23% of men with ED of psychogenic, neurogenic, vasculogenic, and mixed origins, respectively. The median effective dose was 3, 4, 4.5, and 5 µg in the psychogenic, neurogenic, mixed, and vasculogenic groups, respectively. The duration of erection ranged from 11 to 100 minutes (mean, 37 minutes). Penile pain occurred in 34% of men, but only 11% of the total number of injections caused pain.

- *Efficacy and safety study.* Adequate doses of alprostadil (0.2–80 µg) were determined in the clinic for 606 men (89%), and these doses were ≤20 µg in 78%. Four hundred seventy-one men (69%) completed the 6-month trial. Of 13,762 injections after which sexual activity was recorded, 87% resulted in satisfactory sexual activity. Partners rated intercourse as satisfactory on 86% of occasions. Penile pain was reported by 50% of men but after only 11% of injections, indicating that many men had pain only after some injections. Pain was mild in most instances, and only 6% of men withdrew because of pain. Other adverse events (AEs) included prolonged erection (5%), priapism (1%), penile fibrotic complications (2%), and hematoma or ecchymosis (8%).

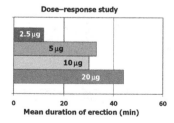
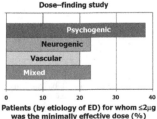

FIGURE 6.2. Efficacy and safety of intracavernous alprostadil in men with erectile dysfunction

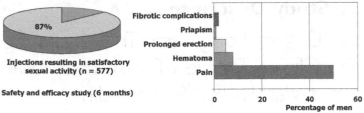

FIGURE 6.2. *Continued*

6.6 CONCLUSIONS FROM ORIGINAL REPORTS
Intracavernosal alprostadil is an effective and tolerable therapy for men with erectile dysfunction, provided that the optimal dose is established individually and that men are trained in the self-injection technique with periodic supervision.

6.7 STRENGTHS
This was a large, multicenter, double-blind, placebo-controlled study in 2 conditions. As such, the overall study design would be difficult to fault, even according to the criteria of 2002. An evaluation of the therapeutic ratio of different doses was also undertaken.

6.8 WEAKNESSES
The report actually represents data from three substudies using similar protocols. However, this does lead to some inconsistencies with respect to inclusion/exclusion criteria and response assessment. There was no long-term follow-up.

6.9 RELEVANCE
This trial supports the findings of the widespread use of PGE_1 in the treatment of ED. The data reflect the clinical experience precisely with respect to responder rate, quality of erection, patient and partner satisfaction, and adverse events.

7. Study Descriptor

An Elegant Long-Term Trial Assessing the Clinical Profile of Intracavernosal Prostaglandin E_1 (Alprostadil)

7.1 KEY TRIAL REFERENCES

7.1.1 Major Publication

Porst H, Buvat J, et al. Intracavernous Alprostadil Alfadex – an effective and well tolerated treatment for erectile dysfunction. Results of a long-term European study. Int J Impot Res 10:225–231, 1998.

7.1.2 Other Important Publications

The long-term safety of alprostadil (prostaglandin – E_1) in patients with erectile dysfunction. The European Alprostadil Study Group. Br J Urol 82(4):538–543, 1998.

Purvis K, Egdetveit I, Christiansen E. Intracavernosal therapy for erectile failure – impact of treatment and reasons for drop-out and dissatisfaction. Int J Impot Res 11(5):287–299, 1999.

7.2 IMPORTANCE OF STUDY

Although by this stage the utility of alprostadil in erectile dysfunction (ED) was well known and the drug was widely used, there had been no long-term analysis of efficacy and safety. This trial showed that efficacy was maintained over a 4-year period and that there was no tachyphylaxis.

7.3 STUDY DESIGN

Prospective, multicenter, long-term study. n = 162.

Following a thorough diagnostic evaluation (medical history, physical examination, and biochemistry), all patients underwent pharmaco-testing with alprostadil (Alfadex). Increasing doses up to 20 μg were used until a rigid erection of >30 minutes, sufficient for intercourse, could be induced. This in-clinic titration was combined with doppler or duplex sonography of the penile vessels to assess arterial inflow.

Erectile response was graded (score 0–3), with score 0 = no response; score 1 = tumescence; score 2 = full tumescence, partial rigidity (erectile angle 45–90°); and score 3 = complete erection (erectile angle >90°). Those patients achieving scores of 2 or 3 were considered responders and were given alprostadil (Alfadex) for self-injection therapy at home. Patients were followed up every 2 to 3 months for 4 years.

7.3.1 Outcome Measures
Penile response to alprostadil (Alfadex) (determined as an erection sufficient for vaginal penetration and the occurrence of sexual intercourse) and the occurrence of side effects were recorded in patient diaries. The diaries were reviewed every 2 months during the first 3 years and then every 3 months during year 4. Annual reviews also included an intracavernous injection of alprostadil (Alfadex) (at the dose used at home) and sonographic assessment.

Subjective assessment of efficacy and tolerability was recorded by questionnaires given to both patients and partners.

7.3.2 Inclusion Criteria
Men with chronic ED (>1 year). The majority of patients had ED of organic etiology (90.7%), and 9.3% were deemed to have ED of purely psychogenic origin. The mean age was 54 years, and the mean duration of ED was 4 years.

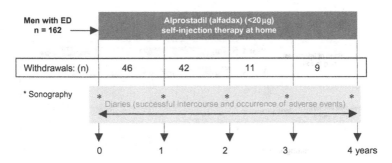

FIGURE 7.1. Alprostadil injection study design

7.4 KEY RESULTS
- The number of injections that resulted in sexual intercourse was 15,713, of a total of 16,886 (93.1%). The number of successful injections (resulting in intercourse) increased from 90.7% in year 1 to 96.3% in year 4.

- Of the 162 patients who were enrolled, 54 completed the 4-year follow-up, giving an overall dropout rate of 66.7%. However, at the end of year 1, three study centers were closed, with the loss of 23 patients. The withdrawal rate from year 2 to the end of year 4 was 33.3%.
- Satisfaction (efficacy and tolerability) was rated as very good to good by 98% of the 54 completers at the end of year 4.
- The incidence of adverse events (AEs) decreased during the course of the study, reflecting patients' increased experience in handling self-injection therapy.
- The incidence of typical AEs associated with self-injection therapy was as follows: Prolonged erections (>6 hours) occurred in 2 patients only during year 1 (1.2%). Painful erections occurred in 29% of patients during year 1 and in 12.1% of patients in year 4. Hematomas (not impeding sexual performance) occurred in 33.3% during year 1, decreasing to 12.1% by year 4. Fibrotic penile changes (nodules, plaques, or deviations) were present in 11.7% of patients overall, with spontaneous healing (on temporary discontinuation of self-injection therapy) occurring in 48% of these patients.
- Comparison of the doppler/duplex examinations for the 54 completers showed an improvement of 25% in blood flow in the deep penile arteries.

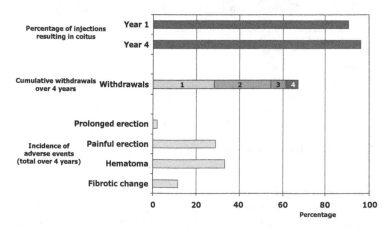

FIGURE 7.2. Long-term efficacy and safety of intracavernous alprostadil (Alfadex) in men with erectile dysfunction

7.5 CONCLUSIONS FROM ORIGINAL REPORTS

The data from this long-term prospective trial provide evidence that self-injection therapy with the vasoactive agent alprostadil (Alfadex) is a very effective and safe treatment of erectile dysfunction of both psychogenic and organic etiologies.

7.6 STRENGTHS

A multicenter study following the clinical response of 162 patients for up to 4 years. Patient characteristics were well defined at baseline.

7.7 WEAKNESSES

As would be expected for any long-term study, few patients (54) reached the 4-year time point, a phenomenon that can complicate interpretation of the data.

7.8 RELEVANCE

This type of study has become almost mandatory in the eyes of the regulatory authorities. The data from this type of study are key for setting appropriate expectations for patients and their partners.

8. Study Descriptor

Evaluation of Novel Combination (Vasoactive Intestinal Polypeptide and Phentolamine) as Intracavernosal Therapy

8.1 KEY TRIAL REFERENCES

8.1.1 Major Publication
Sandhu D, Curless E, et al. A double-blind, placebo controlled study of intracavernosal vasoactive intestinal polypeptide and phentolamine mesylate in a novel auto-injector for the treatment of non-psychogenic erectile dysfunction. Int J Impot Res 11:81–97, 1999.

8.1.2 Other Important Publications
Gerstenberg T, Metz P, et al. Intracavernous self-injection with vasoactive intestinal polypeptide and phentolamine in the management of erectile failure. J Urol 147(5):1277–1279, 1992.

McMahon C. A pilot study of the role on intracavernous injection of vasoactive intestinal polypeptide (VIP) and phentolamine mesylate in the treatment of erectile dysfunction. Int J Impot Res 8(4): 233–236, 1996.

Dinsmore W, Alderdice D. Vasoactive intestinal polypeptide and phentolamine mesylate by autoinjector in the treatment of patients with erectile dysfunction resistant to other intracavernosal agents. Br J Urol 81(3):437–440, 1998.

Dinsmore W, Gingell C, et al. Treating men with predominantly nonpsychogenic erectile dysfunction with intracavernosal vasoactive intestinal polypeptide and phentolamine mesylate in a novel autoinjector system: a multicentre double-blind placebo-controlled study. BJU Int 83(3):274–270, 1999.

8.2 STUDY FUNDING
Senetek plc.

8.3 IMPORTANCE OF STUDY
This trial indicates the potential advantages of using a combination of vasoactive agents. In this case, the combination of

vasoactive intestinal polypeptide (VIP) and phentolamine would appear to offer the advantage of the erection quality of alprostadil in the absence of compliance-limiting pain at the site of injection.

8.4 STUDY DESIGN

Prospective, double-blind, placebo-controlled, crossover study. n = 304.

Dose assessment phase. Erectile response to intracavernosal vasoactive intestinal polypeptide (VIP) 25 µg and phento-lamine 1 mg (VIP/P1), administered by an auto-injector was assessed in the clinic. The injections were administered by the clinician, and visual stimulating material was available as required. A positive response to this test (erection suitable for vaginal penetration) allowed admission to the placebo-controlled phases. Patients failing this test were given auto-injectors for self-administration at home, one containing the VIP/P1 formulation and a second containing 25 µg of VIP and 2 mg of phentolamine (VIP/P2). A positive at home response to either of these injections also allowed entry to the placebo-controlled phases.

Placebo-controlled phases (n = 240). Patients were supplied with two sets of 6 auto-injectors for home use over a 6-month period. Each set of 6 injectors was randomized so that 1 contained placebo and 5 contained active during; the dosages were determined by response during the assessment phase. Patients were instructed to leave at least 36 hours between injections and not to inject more than 3 times per week. At the end of the 6-month period, or following the 12th injection, patients returned to the clinic for review, examination, and dose reassessment. The second placebo-controlled phase was conducted in an identical manner to the first. Successful completion of a phase required a minimum of 9 injections with corresponding diary entries.

8.4.1 Outcome Measures

Dose assessment phase. Erectile response (subjective assessment).

Placebo-controlled phases. Erectile response, duration of response, and adverse events (AEs) were recorded after each injection in patient diaries. The overall satisfaction of patients and their partners was assessed by follow-up questionnaire.

8.4.2. Inclusion Criteria

Men with erectile dysfunction of ≥1 year duration and of non-psychogenic origin.

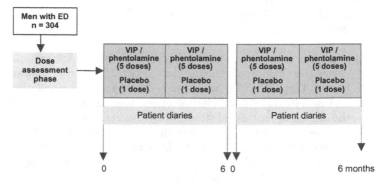

FIGURE 8.1. VIP/phentolamine injection study design

8.5 KEY RESULTS

- During the dose assessment phase, 255/304 patients (83.9%) had an erection suitable for intercourse with either of the 2 doses. Fifteen of these responders withdrew (7 due to AEs and 8 for miscellaneous reasons). In the remaining 289 men, the overall cumulative response rate was 83%. In a subpopulation of 183 men who had withdrawn from previous ED therapies, 82% responded in this trial.
- 195 patients participated in the first placebo-controlled phase, and 133 patients completed this phase. The reasons for withdrawal were AEs (2), noncompliance with protocol (22), withdrawn consent (12), and unknown (26). One hundred twenty-six subjects participated in the second phase, and 105 completed pretrial.
- Overall (both phases), a positive response (erection sufficient for intercourse) was achieved in 1417/1886 injections (75.1%) with VIP/P1 and 45/373 injections (12.1%) with placebo. Similarly for VIP/P2, 257/386 injections (66.5%) resulted in a positive response, compared with 8/78 injections (10.3%) with placebo.
- The median duration of erection with VIP/phentolamine was 54 minutes.

- Differential analysis of active *vs.* placebo response rate by underlying etiology showed that there was no statistically significant difference in the efficacy of VIP/P1 and VIP/P2.
- The principal AE was transient facial flushing, which occurred in 33.9% (placebo 6.9%) of injections. There was no postinjection pain, and there were only 2 episodes of priapism.
- Overall, 85% or more of patients were satisfied or very satisfied with the drug, and more than 95% were satisfied with the injector. More than 81% of patients and 76% of partners considered their quality of life to be improved or greatly improved by the treatment.

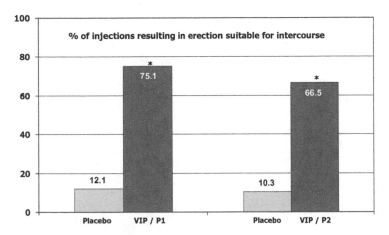

FIGURE 8.2. Efficacy of intracavernosal VIP/phentolamine in men with erectile dysfunction of nonpsychogenic cause (* p < 0.001 vs placebo)

8.6 CONCLUSIONS FROM ORIGINAL REPORTS

These results demonstrate unequivocally that the VIP/phentolamine combination, delivered intracavernosally by auto-injector, is a safe and efficacious treatment for erectile dysfunction of nonpsychogenic origin.

8.7 STRENGTHS

A community-based, double-blind study using a variety of well-established clinical endpoints.

8.8 WEAKNESSES

No direct comparison arm was included in the study design. Comparison with intracavernosal alprostadil would have been desirable.

8.9 RELEVANCE

An excellent study design, likely to be predictive of real-life situations. The data indicate that the combination of VIP/ phentolamine would represent a viable option to intracavernosal alprostadil and may offer advantages over that treatment.

9. Study Descriptor
Now-Classic Study on the Use of Intraurethral Prostaglandin E₁ (Alprostadil)

9.1 KEY TRIAL REFERENCES

9.1.1 Major Publication
Padma-Nathan H, Hellstrom W, et al. Treatment of men with erectile dysfunction with transurethral alprostadil. N Engl J Med 336:1–7, 1997.

9.1.2 Original Abstract
Padma-Nathan H. Treatment of men with erectile dysfunction with transurethral alprostadil. American Urological Association 1996.

9.1.3 Other Important Publications
Engel J, McVary K. Transurethral alprostadil as therapy for patients who withdrew from or failed prior intracavernous injection therapy. Urology 51(5):687–692, 1998.

Fulgham P, Cochran J, et al. Disappointing initial results with transurethral alprostadil for erectile dysfunction in a urology practise setting. J Urol 160 (6 Pt 1):2041–2046, 1998.

9.2 STUDY FUNDING
Vivus, Inc.

9.3 IMPORTANCE OF STUDY
In many ways, this trial illustrates the dangers in the interpretation of early clinical trials data. The many pitfalls for the unwary reader are incorporated into the study design and the subsequent publication. On this basis, alone, it has become a "classic."

9.4 STUDY DESIGN
Randomized, double-blind, placebo-controlled, multicenter prospective study. n = 1511.

Initially the men were tested in the clinic to determine the appropriate dose (125, 250, 500, or 1000 µg) of transurethral alprostadil, administered by the Medicated Urethral System for

Erection (MUSE) system. Penile response to alprostadil was evaluated (score, 1–5) by the patient and confirmed by the investigator. Those men who achieved a maximal response to alprostadil (score 4 or 5) were entered into the 3-month double-blind phase and were randomly assigned to their selected dose or placebo. Patients were evaluated monthly in the clinic.

9.4.1 Outcome Measures
Penile response was assessed by an Erection Assessment Scale: 1 = no response, 2 = some enlargement, 3 = full enlargement (but insufficient rigidity), 4 = erection sufficient for intercourse, and 5 = full rigidity. The duration of response and overall level of comfort were recorded before and 15, 30, 45, and 60 minutes after administration.

During the double-blind phase, the patients and their partners kept diaries documenting penile response, occurrence of intercourse, whether the man achieved orgasm, level of comfort associated with administration, and any adverse events (AEs).

9.4.2 Inclusion Criteria
Men with erectile dysfunction (ED) of primarily organic origin. The age range was 27 to 88 years, and the mean duration of ED was 51 months.

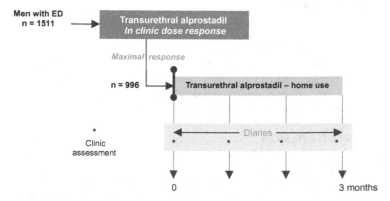

FIGURE 9.1. Transurethral alprostadil (MUSE) study design

9.5 KEY RESULTS

- *In clinic response*. Of the 1511 men, 996 (65.9%) had maximal penile responses (score 4 or 5) with at least one of the doses of alprostadil. The 125-µg dose was selected by 12% of the men, the 250-µg dose by 17%, the 500-µg dose by 30%, and the 100-µg dose by 41%. The proportion of men with maximal response increased with increasing dose. The mean duration of response was also positively correlated with the dose. The transurethral application of alprostadil was rated as neutral, comfortable, or very comfortable by 88% of the men.

- *At-home response*. Of the 996 patients, 961 reported at least one administration, and 873 (87.7%) completed the 3-month period.

- Sexual intercourse was reported to have occurred at least once during the 3-month period by 64.9% of men in the alprostadil group as compared with 18.6% in the placebo group (p < 0.001). Similarly, orgasm was reported by 63.6% of men in the alprostadil group as compared with 23.6% in the placebo group (p < 0.001).

- Among men who reported having sexual intercourse at least once with alprostadil, 7 out of 10 administrations were followed by intercourse.

- Transurethral alprostadil was significantly more effective, regardless of the cause of ED or the age of the patient, when compared with placebo (p > 0.001 for all comparisons). Alprostadil was also more effective than placebo at all dose levels studied.

- The most common side effect of alprostadil was penile pain (usually mild), which was reported by 35.7% of men during in-clinic testing and by 32.7% of men during home treatment (10.8% of home administrations). 2.4% withdrew from the clinic study because of penile pain.

- Hypotension occurred in 3.3% and syncope in 0.4% of men when alprostadil was administered in the clinic. The frequency of hypotension increased with dose from 0.7% with the 125-µg dose to 2.4% in those receiving the 1000-µg dose. Dizziness was reported by 1.9% of alprostadil patients at home, but there was no syncope.

- No incidents of penile fibrosis, urethral stricture, or priapism were reported with the use of transurethral alprostadil.

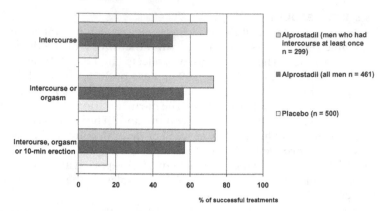

FIGURE 9.2. Efficacy of transurethral alprostadil compared with placebo – home treatment

9.6 CONCLUSIONS FROM ORIGINAL REPORTS
The transurethral administration of alprostadil was well tolerated and effective in restoring the capacity for erections and sexual intercourse in a substantial proportion of men with chronic ED.

9.7 STRENGTHS
This was a large, placebo-controlled, double-blind study of ED, evaluating several doses of intraurethral alprostadil.

9.8 WEAKNESSES
This is a classic example of a "patient-enriched design," in which only patients known to respond to therapy were included in the study.

9.9 RELEVANCE
The claimed response rate (circa 65%) undoubtedly is highly dependent on the patient inclusion/exclusion criteria and is due to population enrichment. A classic marketing study, bearing little relation to likely performance in the community setting.

10. Study Descriptor

Route of Administration Has a Considerable Impact on Clinical Profile: A Comparison of Intraurethral and Intracavernosal Alprostadil

10.1 KEY TRIAL REFERENCES

10.1.1 Major Publication
Porst H. Transurethral alprostadil with MUSE™ (medicated urethral system for erection) vs intracavernous alprostadil – a comparative study in 103 patients with erectile dysfunction. Int J Impot Res 9:187–192, 1997.

10.1.2 Other Important Publications
Shabsigh R, Padma-Nathan H, et al. Intracavernous alprostadil alfadex is more efficacious, better tolerated, and preferred over intraurethral alprostadil plus optional actis: a comparative randomised, crossover, multicentre study. Urology 55(1):109–113, 2000.

10.2 IMPORTANCE OF STUDY
In the field of erectile dysfunction (ED) therapy, few side-by-side comparative studies are carried out. The data from this clinical trial unequivocally show the superiority of intracorporal alprostadil over the intraurethral formulation.

10.3 STUDY DESIGN
Comparative, open label study. n = 103.

In all patients, the effects of intracavernous (i.c.) alprostadil (5–40 µg) were compared with those of transurethral alprostadil with Medicated Urethral System for Erection (MUSE) (125–1000 µg). All administrations and investigations were undertaken by the investigator. The order in which the regimens were given to each patient was randomized.

The start doses were 10 μg (i.c. alprostadil, prostaglandin [PGE_1]) and 500 μg (Alprostadil MUSE), with a minimum of 48 hours washout between administrations. In responders the dosages were lowered to 5 μg PGE_1 and 250 μg MUSE, and in nonresponders the dosages were increased to 20 μg (40 μg in a few cases) or 1000 μg, respectively.

10.3.1 Outcome Measures
Degree of erection: rated from 1 to 5, with responders scoring 4 (full tumescence, partial rigidity) or 5 (full tumescence, full rigidity).

Duplex sonography of penile arteries, to determine the systolic peak low velocities and end-diastolic flow in the deep penile arteries.

Blood pressure (sitting) and occurrence of adverse events (AEs) were monitored for 60 minutes after administration.

At the end of the study, patients were asked which regimen (in terms of efficacy and tolerability) they would prefer for home use.

10.3.2 Inclusion Criteria
Men with ED (>6 months).

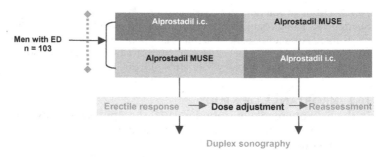

FIGURE 10.1. Intracavernous alprostadil versus intraurethral alprostadil (MUSE) crossover study design

10.4 KEY RESULTS
- The total response rates (score 4 or 5) were 70% with i.c. alprostadil and 43% with alprostadil MUSE. Completely rigid erections (score 5) were obtained in 48% of patients with i.c. alprostadil as compared with 10% with alprostadil MUSE.

- The dosages required to achieve their highest erection score with alprostadil MUSE were 500 µg in 21% of patients and 1000 µg in 56% of patients. For i.c. alprostadil, most patients needed 10 µg (28%) or 20 µg (65%) for their best erection score and 40 µg was required in only 1%.
- At the end of the trial, 37.9% of patients considered i.c. alprostadil superior and 15.5% considered it inferior to MUSE. Some 46.6% of patients indicated that they were not aware of any difference (in terms of efficacy) between the two methods; the majority of these patients were nonresponders.
- The average end-diastolic flow in the deep penile arteries ranged between 9.2 and 9.4 cm/s after MUSE, as compared with 4.5 to 4.8 cm/s after i.c. alprostadil, indicating that a greater degree of relaxation of the cavernous smooth muscle occurred with i.c. alprostadil.
- Penile pain or burning sensation was experienced by 31% of patients with MUSE, as compared with 10.6% with i.c. alprostadil. Urethral bleeding occurred in 4.8% of patients after MUSE administration.
- Clinically relevant systemic AEs (dizziness, sweating, hypotension) occurred in 5.8% of patients after MUSE, with syncope in 1%. No circulatory AEs occured with i.c. alprostadil.

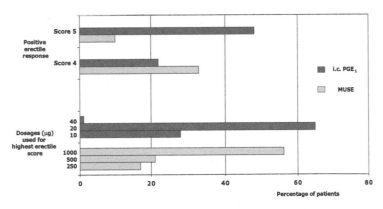

FIGURE 10.2. Efficacy of intracavernous alprostadil (i.c. PGE$_1$) versus transurethral alprostadil (MUSE) in men with erectile dysfunction

10.5 CONCLUSIONS FROM ORIGINAL REPORTS

These results show that i.c. alprostadil has superior efficacy (70% vs. 43%) and fewer side effects than alprostadil MUSE.

Intracavernous injection of alprostadil remains the "gold standard" (in terms of efficacy and reliability) for the pharmacological treatment of erectile dysfunction. MUSE therapy should be reserved for a subset of patients suffering from erectile dysfunction.

10.6 STRENGTHS
All patients were exposed, in a randomized design, to both forms of alprostadil. The clinical investigator is expert in the field of ED management and trial design.

10.7 WEAKNESSES
Endpoints were somewhat subjective, although this does not detract from the conclusions. A dose escalation was used that could result in overestimation of efficacy.

10.8 RELEVANCE
Although the study was conducted in an office setting, the results are likely to be predictive of the relative profiles of intracorporal and intraurethral alprostadil in the community setting. As has become generally acknowledged, intracavernosal alprostadil is the mainstay of self-injection therapy, and intraurethral alprostadil is reserved for a subset of patients.

11. Study Descriptor

First Clinical Data on Sildenafil: The Arrival of Oral Pharmacotherapy

11.1 KEY TRIAL REFERENCES

11.1.1 Major Publication

Boolell M, Allen M, et al. Sildenafil: an orally active type 5 cyclic GMP-specific phosphodiesterase inhibitor for the treatment of penile erectile dysfunction. Int J Impot Res 8:47–52, 1996.

11.1.2 Other Important Publications

Boolell M, Gepi-Attee S, et al. Sildenafil, a novel effective oral therapy for male erectile dysfunction. Br J Urol 78:257–261, 1996.

Olsson A, Speakman M, et al. Sildenafil citrate (Viagra) is effective and well tolerated for treating erectile dysfunction of psychogenic or mixed aetiology. Int J Clin Pract 54(9):561–566, 2000.

Eardley I, Morgan R, et al. Efficacy and safety of sildenafil citrate in the treatment of men with mild to moderate erectile dysfunction. Br J Psychiat 178:325–330, 2001.

11.2 STUDY FUNDING

Pfizer

11.3 IMPORTANCE OF STUDY

This represented the first serious publication indicating the potential utility of sildenafil in the treatment of erectile dysfunction (ED). It represented the arrival of oral therapy for the treatment of ED, offering much hope to patients and physicians alike.

11.4 STUDY DESIGN

Randomized, double-blind, placebo-controlled, four-way crossover study. n = 12.

Patients were administered a single dose of sildenafil (10, 25, or 50 mg) or placebo in a crossover fashion on four different study days. There was a minimum of 3 days between treatments to ensure adequate clearance of sildenafil from the circulation.

On each occasion, visual sexual stimulation (VSS) commenced 30 minutes post-dose and lasted for 2 hours.

11.4.1 Outcome Measures

Erectile response was evaluated by penile plethysmography (Rigiscan) to measure rigidity at the base and tip of the penis.

The primary outcome measure was duration of rigidity >60% at the base and tip of the penis during VSS.

Blood pressure, heart rate, adverse events (AEs), and laboratory safety data were recorded at each study session.

11.4.2 Inclusion Criteria

Men with erectile dysfunction of ≥6 months duration and no obvious organic cause.

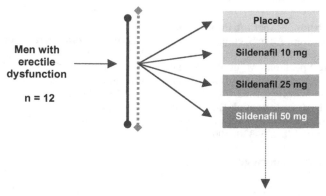

Rigiscan—duration of >60% base and tip penile rigidity during VSS

FIGURE 11.1. Sildenafil versus placebo double blind randomized Rigiscan study design

11.5 KEY RESULTS

- Of the 12 patients, 10 were evaluable.
- The duration of rigidity >60% at the base and tip of the penis during VSS was significantly longer with all doses of sildenafil than with placebo.
- The mean duration of >60% rigidity at the base of the penis was 3.2 minutes with placebo and 25.9, 24.1, and 31.8 minutes with sildenafil at doses of 10, 25, and 50 mg, respectively.

- The mean duration of >60% rigidity at the tip of the penis was 3.0 minutes with placebo and 19.1, 26.3, and 26.5 minutes with sildenafil at doses of 10, 25, and 50 mg, respectively.
- With sildenafil, the onset of penile tumescence was within the initial few minutes of VSS or approximately 30 to 40 minutes post-dosing (corresponding to peak plasma concentrations).
- Mild headache was reported by 4 patients (2 at 25-mg and 2 at 50-mg dosages), which was transient and did not result in withdrawal from the study. There were no significant changes in heart rate, blood pressure, or laboratory clinical data in these patients.

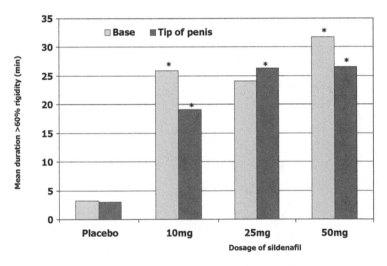

FIGURE 11.2. Efficacy of sildenafil in men with erectile dysfunction of nonorganic cause (*P = 0.0001 vs placebo)

11.6 CONCLUSIONS FROM ORIGINAL REPORTS
These results show that sildenafil enhances the erectile response to VSS in men with ED without any established organic cause.

This highlights the important role of phosphodiesterase type 5 in human penile erection.

11.7 STRENGTHS
Rigorous inclusion and exclusion criteria enabled evaluation to be carried out with a relatively small sample size.

11.8 WEAKNESSES

A relatively small number of patients (12) were evaluated. However, it should be borne in mind that this represented a "proof of concept" study for internal decision making and was not designed as a pivotal regulatory study.

11.9 RELEVANCE

The conclusion of this trial that sildenafil can enhance the erectile response in ED has stood the test of time.

12. Study Descriptor
Original "Gold Standard" Clinical Trial
of Sildenafil in ED

12.1 KEY TRIAL REFERENCES

12.1.1 Major Publication
Goldstein I, Lue T, et al. Oral sildenafil in the treatment of erectile dysfunction. N Engl J Med 338:1397–1404, 1998.

12.1.2 Other Important Publications
Morales A, Gingell C, et al. Clinical safety of oral sildenafil citrate (Viagra) in the treatment of erectile dysfunction. Int J Impot Res 10(2):69–73, 1998.

12.2 STUDY FUNDING
Pfizer

12.3 IMPORTANCE OF STUDY
Although a pilot study had indicated that sildenafil could produce an erectile response in patients with erectile dysfunction (ED), the full clinical potential had not been explored. This trial in patients with ED arising from different etiologies unequivocally demonstrated the benefit in patients with mild to severe ED.

12.4 STUDY DESIGN
Two sequential, multicenter studies. n = 861

Dose-response study. In this double-blind, placebo-controlled, fixed-dose study, 532 men were randomly assigned to placebo or 25, 50, or 100 mg sildenafil for 24 weeks. Patients were instructed to take each dose approximately 1 hour before intercourse and to leave at least a day between doses. Patients' event logs were reviewed at 0, 2, 4, 8, 12, 16, 20, and 24 weeks, and an International Index for Erectile Dysfunction (IIEF) was completed at weeks 0, 12, and 24.

Dose-escalation study with open-label extension. In this flexible dose-escalating study, 329 men were randomly assigned to placebo or 50 mg sildenafil for an initial 12 weeks of treatment. Dosages could be adjusted, depending on therapeutic response and adverse events (AEs), by a 50% reduction or a doubling of the dose, at weeks 2, 4, 8, and 12. All patients completed an IIEF at weeks 0 and 12, and global efficacy was assessed at week 12. Men completing the study were eligible to participate in an open-label extension for an additional 32 weeks.

12.4.1 Outcome Measures

Efficacy was assessed quantitatively by the IIEF questionnaire. The primary outcome measure was the response to question 3 (frequency of penetration) and question 4 (maintenance of erection after penetration); each response was scored from 0 (no attempt at sexual intercourse) to 5 (almost always or always). The five separate response domains of the IIEF were also assessed (erectile function, orgasmic function, sexual desire, intercourse satisfaction, and overall satisfaction). Patient logs and a global efficacy question were also used for qualitative assessment of efficacy.

12.4.2 Inclusion Criteria

Men with erectile dysfunction of ≥6 months duration and of organic (70%), psychogenic (11%), or mixed (18%) origins.

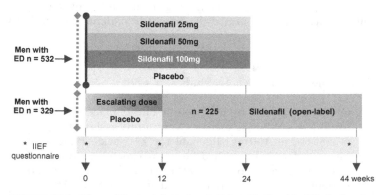

FIGURE 12.1. Phase III pivotal study of sildenafil. Double-blind placebo controlled escalating dose study design

12.5 KEY RESULTS

- *Dose-response study.* Increasing doses of sildenafil were associated with higher mean scores for questions 3 and 4 of the IIEF, and these scores did not vary according to the cause of ED. Scores for the erectile function domain of the IIEF also increased with increasing doses.

- For question 3 (frequency of penetration), the percentage increases in score from baseline to end of treatment were 60%, 84%, and 100% for the 25-, 50-, and 100-mg doses, respectively, compared with 5% for placebo. For question 4 (maintenance of erection), the corresponding values were 121%, 133%, and 130% for the 25-, 50-, and 100-mg groups, compared with 24% for placebo.

- During the last 4 weeks of treatment, the patient logs showed that the proportion of men achieving erections hard enough for sexual intercourse also showed a dose-response relationship: 72%, 80%, and 85% for 25-, 50-, and 100-mg doses of sildenafil, compared with 50% for placebo.

- *Dose-escalation study.* The mean scores for questions 3 and 4 were significantly better with sildenafil than those with placebo after 12 weeks of treatment. For question 3, the score was 95% higher than baseline (placebo 10%) and for question 4, 140% higher (placebo, 13%).

- The mean scores for the erectile function, orgasmic function, intercourse satisfaction, and overall satisfaction domains of the IIEF were significantly higher for sildenafil than for placebo. The mean score for the sexual desire domain was not significantly different from that with placebo.

- During the last 4 weeks of treatment, 69% of all attempts at intercourse were successful, as compared with 22% with placebo, and the mean number of successful attempts was 5.9 for sildenafil and 1.5 for placebo.

- *Open label-extension.* The additional 32 weeks of treatment were completed by 92% of patients, and withdrawals due to treatment-related AEs occurred in 2%.

- *Adverse events.* The most common AEs with sildenafil in the dose-response and dose-escalation studies, respectively, were headache (22% and 18%), flushing (19% and 18%), and dyspepsia (9% and 6%). Withdrawals due to treatment-related AEs occurred in 1% of all sildenafil patients (both studies).

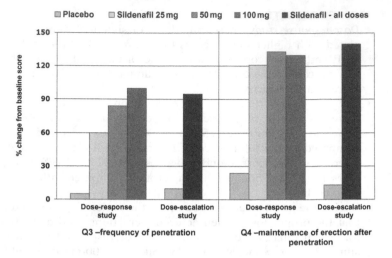

FIGURE 12.2. Efficacy of sildenafil in men with erectile dysfunction of various causes (determined by change in scores for questions 3 and 4 of the IIEF)

12.6 CONCLUSIONS FROM ORIGINAL REPORTS
Sildenafil is an effective, reliable, and well tolerated treatment for men with ED of various etiologies.

The data show that sildenafil was effective in improving erectile function (frequency of penetration and maintenance of erection after penetration) and quadrupled the success of intercourse, with effectiveness maintained for at least 6 months.

12.7 STRENGTHS
Placebo-controlled study of reasonable duration (24 weeks) incorporating, in part, an open-label extension. The newly validated International Index of Erectile Function (IIEF) was used to define more objectively the clinical endpoints that had been possible in earlier studies.

12.8 WEAKNESSES
The dose-escalation design is known to result in overestimation of efficacy (responder rate).

12.9 RELEVANCE
Overall, this trial was predictive of the clinically effective dose range of sildenafil, the spectrum of effect (types of ED patients), the response versus severity of ED, and the tolerability of the drug.

13. Study Descriptor

Pilot Study Showing Benefit of Clinical Response to Apomorphine Sublingual (SL)

13.1 KEY TRIAL REFERENCES

13.1.1 Major Publication

Heaton J, Morales A, et al. Recovery of erectile function by the oral administration of apomorphine. Urology 45(2):200–206, 1995.

13.1.2 Other Important Publications

Dula E, Bukofzer S, et al. Double-blind, crossover comparison of 3 mg apomorphine SL with placebo and 4 mg apomorphine in male erectile dysfunction. Eur Urol 39:558–564, 2001.

Heaton J. Key issues from the clinical trials of apomorphine SL. World J Urol 19(1):25–31, 2001.

Heaton J, Altwein J. The role of apomorphine SL in the treatment of male erectile dysfunction. BJU Int 88(Suppl 3):36–38, 2001.

13.2 STUDY FUNDING

Medical Research Council of Canada, Pharmaceutical Manufacturers of Canada, Pentech Pharmaceuticals

13.3 IMPORTANCE OF STUDY

This study became the foundation of the development program culminating in the approval of apomorphine SL for the treatment of erectile dysfunction (ED). Using this formulation, the Canadian group showed that the benefit of apomorphine, i.e., a good erectile response, can be achieved in the absence of compliance-limiting side effects.

13.4 STUDY DESIGN

A four-phase, single-blind, placebo-controlled, dose-escalating study. n = 2–12.

Patients were thoroughly assessed to establish the etiology of their ED, and only patients with ED of psychogenic origin were included. The four phases of this study evaluated the erectile response to and tolerability of four different formulations of apomorphine.

In all phases, patients were tested on at least 3 separate study days, with at least 3 days between. On each test day a single dose was used, and patients were given increasing doses with each testing. Domperidone was used as a pretreatment if nausea had occurred at the previous dose level. The following dosages were used:

Phase 1: placebo: 10 and 20 mg apomorphine (sublingual solution)
Phase 2: placebo: 2.5 and 5 mg apomorphine (sublingual tablet)
Phase 3: 1.25 mg/puff apomorphine (nasal spray)
Phase 4: placebo: 3, 4, and 5 mg apomorphine (controlled-release sublingual tablet)

Erectile response to the drug during visual erotic and sexually neutral stimulation was determined by Rigiscan monitoring.

13.4.1 Outcome Measures

Erectile response: Rigiscan measurements were expressed as a single score (Rigiscan number [RN], range 0–36) to describe changes in circumference, rigidity, and duration; a score of ≥ 16 was considered to be suitable for intercourse. The erectile response to the neutral video was calculated as the percentage of the response to the preceding erotic video to ascertain the effects of apomorphine alone.

Visual analogue scales (VAS) were used before and after drug administration to assess the patient's senses of well-being, tranquillity, anxiety, and arousal, their level of sedation, and changes in yawning behavior. Blood pressure (BP) and heart rate (HR) were also recorded at the start and finish of each session. Adverse events were recorded by spontaneous reporting.

13.4.2 Inclusion Criteria

Men with erectile dysfunction of psychogenic origin.

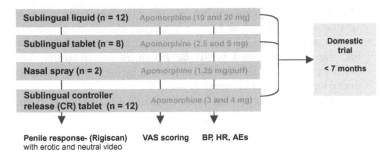

FIGURE 13.1. Study design of placebo controlled multiple delivery system study of apomorphine

13.5 KEY RESULTS

- *Phase 1.* Of the 10 evaluable patients, 7 were complete responders to apomorphine SL solution, with an RN ≥16 for both erotic and neutral video segments. Six of these patients continued with apomorphine in a domestic trial (duration, 2–7 months), and 3 of them required domperidone pretreatment.
- Analysis of the VAS scoring indicated that patients were relaxed, not sedated, and without sexual arousal or anxiety. AEs were reported at both doses of apomorphine. Eight patients experienced typical side effects of unmodified apomorphine administration (sudden nausea, diaphoresis, dizziness, pallor, visual disturbances, hypotension, and bradycardia), varying in duration from 1 to 40 minutes.
- *Phase 2.* Of the 7 evaluable patients, 2 were responders (score ≥ 16), and both successfully used apomorphine SL tablets at the lower dose (2.5 mg) in a domestic trial for no less than 2 months. The 5-mg tablets were associated with the same significant side effects as the apomorphine solution.
- *Phase 3.* Only 2 patients were administered apomorphine by intranasal spray, and both experienced significant AEs (yawning, nausea, vomiting, dizziness, blurred vision, diaphoresis, pallor, hypotension, and bradycardia). No further attempts were made to test this preparation.
- *Phase 4.* Of 12 patients, 8 successfully developed erections after administration of apomorphine CR, SL tablets. Both the 3-mg and the 4-mg doses produced an excellent response, with a significant increase in the RN for erotic and neutral video segments, and comparison of these scores indicated that 70%–80% of an apomorphine-aided erotic erection will be

obtained with apomorphine alone. The VAS scoring was similar to that in phase 1.

- At the doses tested, this preparation was devoid of AEs that had been experienced with the previous preparations. The primary effect of yawning was reported, but at a lower number and frequency than previously seen.
- Home use was successful and sustained in 7 of 11 patients (64%).

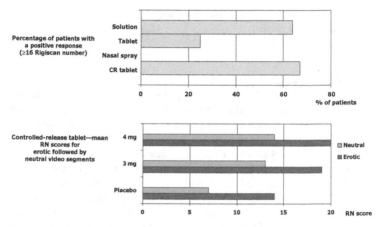

FIGURE 13.2. Erectile response to different formulations of apomorphine

13.6 CONCLUSIONS FROM ORIGINAL REPORTS

These results show that apomorphine will act as an erectogenic agent when absorbed through the oral mucosa.

Apomorphine SL (controlled absorption, 3 or 4 mg) will cause durable erections without side effects in 67% of men who have no documentable organic cause of their ED.

13.7 STRENGTHS

This pilot study, although small, was conducted under rigorous conditions by a group experienced in clinical trial design, drug development, and the management of ED.

13.8 WEAKNESSES

As expected for a pilot or "proof of concept" study, the number of patients was relatively small.

13.9 RELEVANCE

The findings of this pilot study have been confirmed in considerably more extensive studies as part of the successful registration program for apomorphine SL. The drug has been shown to be effective in up to 70% of patients, and the benefit is maintained in the long term. Over the effective dose range, the drug is well tolerated.

14. Study Descriptor

A Viable Alternative to PDE Inhibitors: Definition of Therapeutic Ratio of Apomorphine Sublingual (SL) in Patients with ED

14.1 KEY TRIAL REFERENCES

14.1.1 Major Publication
Dula E, Bukofzer S, et al. Double-blind, crossover comparison of 3 mg apomorphine SL with placebo and 4 mg apomorphine in male erectile dysfunction. Eur Urol 39:558–564, 2001.

14.1.2 Other Important Publications
Altwein J, Keuler F. Oral treatment of erectile dysfunction with apomorphine SL. Urol Int 67(4):257–263, 2001.

Mulhall J, Bukofzer S, et al. An open-label, uncontrolled dose-optimising study of sublingual apomorphine in erectile dysfunction. Clin Ther 23(8):1260–1271, 2001.

Fagan T, Buttler S, et al. Cardiovascular safety of sublingual apomorphine in patients on stable doses of oral antihypertensive agents and nitrates. Am J Cardiol 1;88(7):760–766, 2001.

14.2 STUDY FUNDING
TAP Pharmaceutical Products, Inc.

14.3 IMPORTANCE OF STUDY
Apomorphine SL, a dopamine agonist, offers an alternative to phosphodiesterase inhibitors. In any drug development program, it is important to evaluate a range of doses to determine the risk-benefit ratio. This trial showed that the efficacy of apomorphine 3 mg was substantially better than that of placebo. The 4-mg dose offered only equivalent efficacy, but tolerability was reduced. This led to the selection of a top dose of 3 mg apomorphine SL.

14.4 STUDY DESIGN
Randomized, double-blind, crossover, multicenter study. n = 296.

This study included two separate patient groups comparing 3 mg apomorphine SL with placebo (n = 194) and 3 mg apomorphine SL with the 4-mg dosage (n = 102). The trial consisted of two 4-week crossover treatment periods with a 24- to 96-hour washout between.

The presence and severity of ED was established at baseline by using the erectile function domain of the International Index for Erectile Dysfunction (IIEF), and partner perception of ED was assessed by using the Brief Sexual Function Index (BSFI). The initial dose of apomorphine was taken in the clinic, and the patients were observed for 2 hours subsequently. Prochlorperazine (5 mg) was supplied on request. All patients agreed to make a minimum of 2 attempts at sexual intercourse per week and to allow at least 8 hours between doses. Patients were reviewed in the clinic at the beginning and end of each treatment period.

14.4.1 Outcome Measures

The primary efficacy variable was the number of attempts resulting in erections firm enough for intercourse. Time to erection and the occurrence of intercourse were also recorded in patient/partner diaries. Adverse events (AEs) were recorded by direct questioning and spontaneous reporting in diaries.

14.4.2 Inclusion Criteria

Men with erectile dysfunction (inability to attain and maintain an erection firm enough for intercourse in >50% of attempts), of various etiologies and of ≥3 months duration.

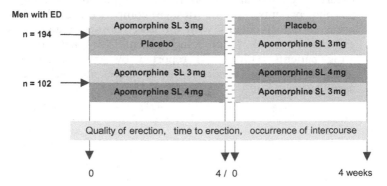

FIGURE 14.1. Pivotal, phase III, placebo controlled double-blind study of Apomorphine SL at variable doses: study design

14.5 KEY RESULTS

- *Apomorphine SL 3 mg vs. placebo.* Apomorphine SL 3 mg resulted in significantly more erections firm enough for intercourse than placebo (46.9% vs. 32.3%, p < 0.001). The partners' assessment of this variable supported that of the patients. Apomorphine SL 3 mg was also superior to placebo for the proportion of attempts resulting in sexual intercourse (patient assessment: 48% vs. 34%, p < 0.001). The average median time to erection was 18.8 minutes for apomorphine.
- In both the placebo and the apomorphine groups, erectile function (IIEF domain) was improved from baseline, but the difference in improvement between the 2 groups was statistically significant (30.3% vs. 4.1%, p < 0.001). Similarly, the improvement in the intercourse satisfaction domain was significantly better with apomorphine (27.8% vs. 11.8%).
- Subgroup analyses by baseline ED severity showed apomorphine SL to be superior to placebo across all severities and comorbidities for the primary efficacy variable.
- *Apomorphine SL 3 mg vs. 4 mg.* There were no statistically significant differences between the two doses of apomorphine for primary and secondary efficacy variables. The proportion of attempts resulting in erections firm enough for intercourse was 49% and 50% for the 3-mg and 4-mg doses, respectively. Similarly, intercourse occurred in 48% and 50% of attempts.
- Subgroup analyses by baseline ED severity and comorbidity showed no meaningful differences between the two doses.
- *Adverse events.* The most common AE was nausea, which was reported by 7% of apomorphine SL 3-mg patients vs. 1.1% of placebo patients. In the dosage comparison study, AEs occurred less frequently with the lower dosage; nausea was experienced by 3.3% of 3-mg patients vs. 14.1% of the 4-mg patients. Other AEs reported by ≥5% of patients included yawning, dizziness, somnolence, headache, and vasodilation.

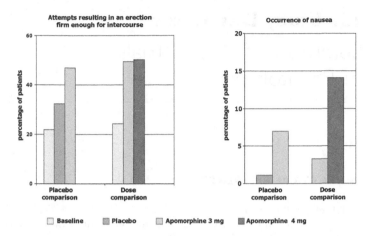

FIGURE 14.2. Efficacy and tolerability of apomorphine SL (3 mg) compared with placebo and apomorphine SL (4 mg) in men with erectile dysfunction

14.6 CONCLUSIONS FROM ORIGINAL REPORTS

Apomorphine SL 3 mg was significantly more effective than placebo in the treatment of men with ED of various etiologies. It had a relatively rapid onset of action (18.8 minutes), allowing for sexual spontaneity, and had an acceptable safety profile.

The 3-mg dose was comparable to the 4-mg dose in terms of efficacy but offered an improved risk-benefit ratio.

14.7 STRENGTHS

A randomized, double-blind, crossover study, assessing efficacy and safety. Patients with ED arising from a wide variety of etiologies were evaluated. The validated International Index of Erectile Function (IIEF) was used, and patient and partner satisfaction was determined.

14.8 WEAKNESSES

No attempt was made to measure penile tumescence and rigidity using, for example, Rigiscan.

14.9 RELEVANCE

In larger clinical trials and from extensive postmarketing experience, apomorphine SL (2 and 3 mg) has been shown to be safe and effective. It has been a most welcome addition to the physician's armamentarium against ED.

15. Study Descriptor
Summary of Clinical Trials of Phentolamine

15.1 KEY TRIAL REFERENCES

15.1.1 Major Publication
Goldstein I, Carson C, et al. Vasomax for the treatment of male erectile dysfunction. World J Urol 19:51–56, 2001.

15.1.2 Other Important Publications
Goldstein I. Oral phentolamine: an alpha-1, alpha-2 adrenergic antagonist for the treatment of erectile dysfunction. Int J Impot Res 12(suppl 1):S75–80, 2000.

15.2 IMPORTANCE OF STUDY
Although it represents a composite of more than one clinical study, this work helps to define the potential of phentolamine in the management of erectile dysfunction (ED). The use of oral (buccal) phentolamine could represent a viable alternative to phospho diesterase (PDE) inhibitors or for use in sildenafil failures.

15.3 STUDY DESIGN
ZON 303 – parallel group, open-label, long-term study. n = 2003.

All patients received an initial test dose of 40 mg oral phentolamine (Vasomax), and 1927 patients then underwent 4 weeks of treatment (taken on an "as needed" basis) at this dose level. Seven hundred twenty-seven of these patients then received an 80-mg test dose, and 691 patients were titrated up to the 80-mg dose for home treatment. Patients then proceeded to 12 months of treatment in these two parallel groups (40 mg and 80 mg), with follow-up visits at 1, 2, 6, and 12/13 months.

15.3.1 Outcome Measures
The primary efficacy endpoint was a change from baseline in the erectile function (EF) domain score (0–30) of the International Index for Erectile Dysfunction (IIEF).

15.3.2 Inclusion Criteria

Men with mild to moderate erectile dysfunction of predominantly organic or mixed origin.

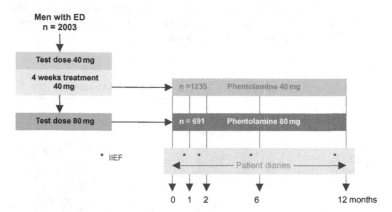

FIGURE 15.1. Escalating doses of oral (buccal) phentolamine for ED: design of studies

15.4 KEY RESULTS

- Patients taking either the 40-mg or the 80-mg dose of phentolamine showed clinically meaningful improvement from baseline in the EF domain of the IIEF.
- These improvements increased in a time-dependent fashion from 1 to 6 months and were sustained at 12 months.
- For the 40-mg dosage, the baseline EF domain score was 17.6 and it increased by 4.9, 6.13, 6.87, and 6.32 points at 1, 2, 6, and 12 months, respectively.
- For the 80-mg dosage, the baseline EF domain score was 17.1, and it changed by −1.05, +4.82, +6.02, and +5.66 points at 1, 2, 6, and 12 months, respectively.
- The attrition rate was high with n = 1522, 1021, 570, and 351 at 1, 2, 6, and 12 months, respectively. Most dropouts were not due to adverse events on lack of efficacy. Sildenafil was approved during the course of the study, and many patients elected to join other trials. Patients who remained in the study showed high levels of treatment efficacy up to 2 years.
- Safety data for this long-term study are not presented in this publication. However, in two previous placebo-controlled, 4-week studies, the adverse events rates were 25% for the 40-mg

group and 42% for the 80-mg group, compared with 17% for placebo. The most common adverse events (AEs) in all phentolamine-treated patients were nasal congestion (10%), headache (3%), dizziness (3%), tachycardia (3%), and nausea (91%). There was a dose relationship for cardiovascular AEs, with comparative incidences for the 40-mg and 80-mg groups of 1.5% vs. 7% for tachycarchia, 0.6% vs 1.5% for palpitations, and 0.2% vs 2.0% for hypotension.

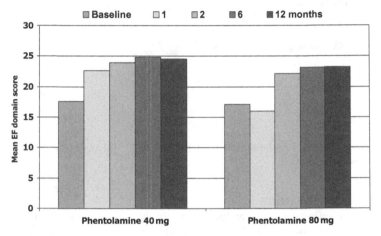

FIGURE 15.2. Long-term efficacy of oral phentolamine (Vasomax) in men with erectile dysfunction of organic or mixed causes (determined by change in erectile function domain score of IIEF)

15.5 CONCLUSIONS FROM ORIGINAL REPORTS
Oral phentolamine mesylate (Vasomax) appears to be effective in the treatment of ED of organic and mixed etiologies. Improvements in EF were seen up to 6 months and were sustained after 12 months of treatment. The drug was well tolerated by the majority of patients, with a satisfactory side effects profile and without significant risk of cardiovascular effects.

15.6 STRENGTHS
A wide range of placebo-controlled and open-label extension studies are described. Over 4000 patients were evaluated, indicating that the clinical database was equivalent to that for sildenafil at the time of submission for regulatory approval.

15.7 WEAKNESSES

Overall, many of the effects of phentolamine are modest.

15.8 RELEVANCE

The data would indicate phentolamine could make an important contribution to patient treatment. The drug at the recommended doses (40 and 80 mg) has an excellent safety profile, and it would afford clinically significant improvement beyond placebo.

16. Study Descriptor
Impact of Testosterone Replacement
in Androgen-Deficient Males

16.1 KEY TRIAL REFERENCES

16.1.1 Major Publication
Skakkebaek N, Bancroft J, et al. Androgen replacement with oral testosterone undecanoate in hypogonadal men: a double-blind controlled study. Clin Endocrinol 14:49–61, 1981.

16.1.2 Other Important Publications
O'Carroll R, Bancroft J. Testosterone therapy for low sexual interest and erectile dysfunction in men: a controlled study. Br J Psychiat 145:146–151, 1984.

Gooren L. A ten-year safety study of the oral androgen testosterone undecanoate. J Androl 15(3):212–215, 1994.

Morales A, Johnston B, et al. Testosterone supplementation for hypogonadal impotence: assessment of biochemical measures and therapeutic outcomes. J Urol 157(3):849–854, 1997.

16.2 STUDY FUNDING
Organon International, Danish Medical Research Council.

16.3 IMPORTANCE OF STUDY
The first carefully controlled study showing the benefit of androgen replacement given to androgen-deficient males.

16.4 STUDY DESIGN
A double-blind, placebo-controlled crossover study. n = 12.

The study group was composed of 6 hypergonadotropic men and 6 hypogonadotropic men, who were balanced between two treatment groups. The subjects were assessed for 1 month while receiving their previous androgen treatment and for 2 months with no treatment. The subjects then received either 160 mg testosterone undecanoate (TU) daily (in 2 doses, 12 hours apart) or placebo for 2 months, followed by 2 months on the other regimen.

16.4.1 Outcome Measures

Diaries were kept throughout the study period, recording sexual acts (intercourse masturbation), occurrence of ejaculation, and subjective quality of the sexual act (1 = unpleasant to 4 = very satisfactory). The men also made weekly ratings of frequency of sexual thoughts and the extent to which those thoughts were associated with sexual excitement and mood (Lorr and McNair Mood Check List), giving scales for anxiety/tension, depression, anger, vigor and fatigue.

At monthly interviews, the investigator rated the patient's enjoyment of sexual contact and his erectile and ejaculatory difficulties. Blood was also collected monthly for endocrine assessment (testosterone, 5 α-dihydrotestosterone, estradiol, sex hormone-binding globulin [SHBG], FSH, LH, and prolactin).

16.4.2 Inclusion Criteria

Androgen-deficient men; in hypergonadotropic men due to castration or primary testicular failure and in hypogonadotropic men due to hypothalamic or pituitary deficiency.

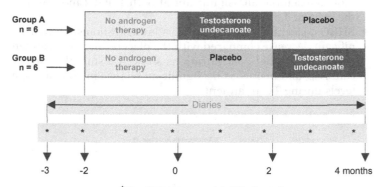

* Investigator assessment and blood sampling

FIGURE 16.1. Placebo controlled, double-blind crossover study of testosterone undecanoate: study design

16.5 KEY RESULTS

- The two diagnostic groups were similar in their response to TU. Although the numbers were too small, there was no indication that hypergonadotropic patients responded better than hypogonadotropic patients.
- Analysis of behavioral scores excluded the first–2–2 weeks of each treatment period in order to minimize the carryover effects of testosterone into the placebo period.

- In all the sexual behavior variables, both those assessed by the investigator and those assessed by the patient, and self-rated (except subjective quality of sexual intercourse), there was a highly significant difference in favor of TU.
- The weekly number of sexual acts for all men increased from 0.8 in the no-treatment period to 2.1 with TU (placebo, 0.7). Similarly, the number of ejaculations per week increased from 0.3 with no treatment to 1.7 with TU (placebo, 0.2).
- Sexual interest (frequency of sexual thoughts and excitement) tended to increase within the first week of androgen replacement, and ejaculation started to return at 2 weeks.
- Testosterone concentrations measured at 0 hours, predose, and 4 hours, postdose, were significantly increased during TU treatment compared with the "no-treatment" levels. The postdose testosterone concentration was also highly significantly different from placebo at both 1 month and 2 months. However, this modest rise in testosterone concentrations did not reach normal range in 4 subjects.
- Increases in 5 α-dihydrotestosterone concentrations were more substantial and significant at both 1 and 2 months after the start of TU treatment.
- SHBG concentrations during TU administration showed a significant decrease compared with the placebo and no-treatment periods. Estradiol concentrations showed a small but significant rise, and there was no significant change in gonadotropin levels during TU treatment.

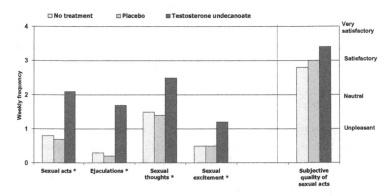

FIGURE 16.2. Treatment response (self-reported) to testosterone undecanoate in hypogonadai men compared with placebo (*significant for active treatment)

16.6 CONCLUSIONS FROM ORIGINAL REPORTS

The behavioral response to testosterone undecanoate was good and fairly rapid, suggesting that lower doses of testosterone are required to maintain sexual behavior than are normally present, or that the behavioral effects are more dependent on the rise in 5 α-dihydrotestosterone.

These results suggest that androgens are necessary for normal male sexuality, although the amount and type of androgens required still need to be clarified.

16.7 STRENGTHS

Remarkably for this era, a carefully controlled, double-blind, placebo-controlled, crossover study. Highly relevant clinical endpoints were employed for the assessment of general and sexual behaviors.

16.8 WEAKNESSES

Only 6 patients per group were studied, encompassing androgen deficiency arising from many different endocrine backgrounds.

16.9 RELEVANCE

This study provides a rational basis for the use of androgen replacement in sexual dysfunction secondary to androgen deficiency across a wide range of etiologies. It cannot be used in support of androgens in the treatment of the "andropause."

17. Study Descriptor
Evaluation of Psychotherapy for
Patients and Partners

17.1 KEY TRIAL REFERENCES

17.1.1 Major Publication
Wylie K. Treatment outcome of brief couple therapy in psychogenic male
erectile disorder. Arch Sexual Behav 26(5): 527–45, 1997.

17.1.2 Other Important Publications
Wylie K. Male erectile disorder; characteristics and treatment choice of
a longitudinal cohort study of men. Int J Impot Res 9(4):217–224,
1997.

Baum N, Randrup E, et al. Prostaglandin E_1 versus sex therapy in the
management of psychogenic erectile dysfunction. Int J Impot Res
12(3):191–194, 2000.

McCarthy B. Relapse prevention strategies and techniques with erectile
dysfunction. J Sex Marital Ther 27(1):1–8, 2001.

17.2 IMPORTANCE OF STUDY
One of the first and best studies of the quantification of the
effects of psychotherapy on patients with erectile dysfunction
(ED). In comparison with baseline, couples continuing therapy
had a positive outcome.

17.3 STUDY DESIGN
Prospective, interventional study. n = 37 couples.

Patients were initially offered a range of treatments: sex
therapy (individual or couple), oral medications (yohimbine or an
investigational drug), intracavernous injections, or vacuum constriction devices. Those couples accepting couple therapy were
entered into this study approximately 3 weeks after initial assessment. During this pretreatment period, diaries were kept recording sexual interest, presence of erections, and attempts at sexual
intercourse. These diaries were repeated at the end of therapy.

The couple therapy package included Modified Modern Sex
Therapy (MMST) and Behavioral Systems Couple Therapy

(BSCT). Six therapy sessions were provided at fortnightly intervals, and failure to progress in relationship therapy or noncompletion of sex therapy homework assignments by the third session resulted in systemic interventions being used (Crowe and Ridley hierarchy).

17.3.1 Outcome Measures
Relationship satisfaction was recorded by using the Golombok Rust Inventory of Marital State (GRIMS). Sexual satisfaction was recorded by using the Golombok Rust Inventory of Sexual Satisfaction (GRISS) and the Pleasant/Unpleasant Feelings questionnaire.

Two target symptoms were also identified and assessed on a 12-point scale: Symptom A, "difficulty in attaining or maintaining an erection," and symptom B, "lack of enjoyment from our sexual relationship."

Global change in the couple's sexual and general relationship was rated by the investigator at the end of therapy. The patient's emotional sate was evaluated by the Hospital Anxiety Depression scale (HAD).

17.3.2 Inclusion Criteria
Men (aged 18–70 years) with ED of psychogenic or combined etiologies (5 patients), in whom erectile failure was present for >3 months and occurred in more than 50% of coital attempts.

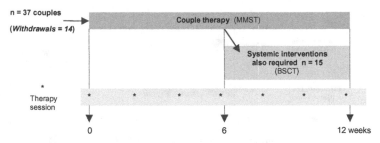

FIGURE 17.1. Couples therapy for ED: study design

17.4 KEY RESULTS
- Of the 23 couples completing therapy, 15 couples required "systems" as well as behavioral interventions.
- With regard to relationship satisfaction, there were no significant changes in the mean GRIMS score before and after therapy.

- Statistically significant improvements in sexual satisfaction (total GRISS score) for men were recorded, and a decrease in the difference of the couples' scores was noted.
- Significant improvements were also noted in men for impotence and infrequency of sexual activity GRISS subscores. Partners also reported a reduction in infrequency of sexual activity, although this was not significant. Similarly, both partners reported a reduction in noncommunication subscore, but reaching statistical significance only in men. Men also reported a significant reduction in the avoidance of sexual activity.
- For target symptom A ("difficulty in attaining or maintaining an erection"), significant improvements were reported by both men and their partners.
- For target symptom B ("lack of enjoyment from our sexual relationship"), improvement was also reported by both men, and their partners, but the change was statistically significant only in men.
- Pre- and post-treatment diaries were completed by 20 men, and these showed a significant increases in the active erection score and in attempts at sexual activity. No changes were reported for interest in sex, number of days with an erection, and spontaneous erections.
- Global outcome: in the 23 couples completing therapy, the outcome was considered to be excellent in 10 couples, moderate in 4, and mild in 6. The remaining 3 couples were considered to show no change or to be worse than at initial assessment.

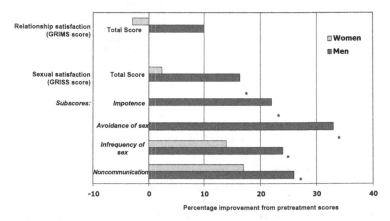

FIGURE 17.2. Changes in psychological scores for couples completing brief couple therapy for male erectile disorder (*significant improvement)

17.5 CONCLUSIONS FROM ORIGINAL REPORTS

This study demonstrates the beneficial outcome of brief couple therapy combining behavioral-systems couple therapy (BSCT) and modified modern sex therapy (MMST) for men with psychogenic factors associated with ED.

17.6 STRENGTHS

Study undertaken in a world-class ED center by an expert psychotherapist/community healthcare physician.

17.7 WEAKNESSES

Almost inevitably with psychometric evaluations, scoring systems cannot be directly related to changes in sexual activity. Analysis is performed only in a clinically defined subpopulation. Perhaps for ethical reasons, there is no placebo control (e.g., equivalent sessions where general rather than relationship dialogue took place).

17.8 RELEVANCE

There is no doubt that there is a positive treatment outcome as compared with baseline. The magnitude of the effect (in the absence of a placebo group) remains unknown. Unquestionably, however, the study shows that patients and couples will gain benefit from extra contact with experienced healthcare providers.

18. Study Descriptor

Quantification of Benefit of a Vacuum Device on Erectile Function

18.1 KEY TRIAL REFERENCES

18.1.1 Major Publication
Bosshardt R, Farwerk R, et al. Objective measurement of the effectiveness, therapeutic success and dynamic mechanisms of the vacuum device. Br J Urol 75:786–791, 1995.

18.1.2 Other Important Publications
Opsomer R, Wese F, et al. The external vacuum device in the management of erectile dysfunction. Acta Urol Belg 65(4):13–16, 1997.

Soderdahl D, Thrasher J, Hansberry K. Intracavernosal drug-induced erection therapy versus external vacuum devices in the treatment of erectile dysfunction. Br J Urol 79(6):952–957, 1997.

Chen J, Mabjeesh N, Greenstein A. Sildenafil versus the vacuum device: patient preference. J Urol 166(5):1779–1781, 2001

18.2 IMPORTANCE OF STUDY
This represents the first attempt at the quantification of the response of the erectile dysfunction (ED) patient to a vacuum device. The study provides evidence that a vacuum device, preferably in conjunction with a constriction ring, will provide some degree of clinical benefit.

18.3 STUDY DESIGN
Open-label study. n = 30.

Men entered into the trial following a 2-week period of home use with the vacuum device (VD). Patients underwent thorough evaluation, including prostaglandin E_1 (PGE_1) injection, doppler sonographic measurement of penile arterial blood flow, nocturnal penile tumescence rigidity (NPTR), and questionnaire.

Tumescence and rigidity of the flaccid penis were recorded by Rigiscan real time monitoring (RTM) for 10 minutes. Following use of the VD and placement of the constriction ring, Rigiscan monitoring was repeated for 20 minutes for the penis in the erect state. Subsequently, all patients performed three NPTRs using Rigiscan at home. The RTM recordings, NPTRs, and questionnaires were repeated after 6 months of home use of the VD.

Intracavernous pressure measurements for the erect penis following use of the VD were made in 13 randomly selected patients. Blood gas analysis (BGA) was also performed in 12 patients to calculate the proportional contribution of venous and arterial cavernous blood immediately after application of the VD and constriction ring and again at 15 and 30 minutes (with the ring still in place).

18.3.1 Outcome Measures
Change in penile rigidity (base and tip) with the use of the VD was determined by the Rigiscan monitor. Changes in the duration and extent of NPTR were assessed before and after treatment. Intracavernous pressure and BGA after use of VD was also determined. An efficacy questionnaire for the VD was completed pretreatment and at the 6-month follow-up.

18.3.2 Inclusion Criteria
Men with erectile dysfunction; the age range was 46–76, years with a mean duration of impotence of 6.6 years. The etiology of erectile dysfunction was diagnosed as vascular in 10 patients, neurological in 4, mixed (neurological/vascular) in 13, and psychological in 3.

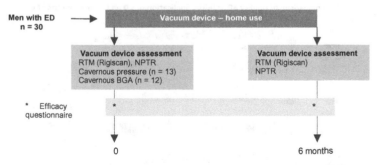

FIGURE 18.1. Vacuum device (VD) effectiveness and usage: study design

18.4 KEY RESULTS
• Four patients were lost to follow-up. The 26 men who completed the study were able to have sexual intercourse after using the VD. The average frequency on intercourse was twice a week for those 23 men who had a partner.

- At the initial assessment of the VD, the average rigidity was 79% at the base and 62% at the tip. These values increased to 84% and 81%, respectively, after 6 months, although the change was significant only for tip rigidity (p < 0.01).
- Mean penile tumescence also increased after 6 months from 3.4 to 3.8 cm at the base and from 2.2 to 2.6 cm at the tip. This increase was not significant.
- After 6 months, the mean NPTR improved, but not significantly. The only NPTR variable to show significant improvement was the duration of the best erectile event measured at the tip.
- However, in the subset of patients reporting spontaneous morning erections (n = 15), there were significant improvements in the following NPTR variables: mean total duration of erection, duration of best erectile event, plateau phase at the base, tumescence increase at the tip, and mean effective rigidity.
- BGA of the cavernous blood determined 30 minutes after application of the constriction ring showed ischemia of the penile blood, and the mean contribution of arterial and venous blood was 58% and 42%, respectively. The mean increase in penis volume was 85 ml.
- For the 13 patients in whom intracavernous pressure was determined, there was a correlation between basal rigidity and intracavernous pressure.

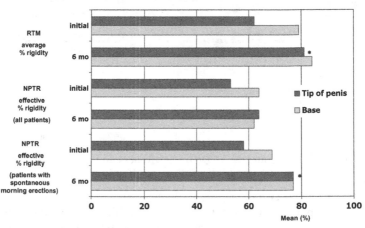

FIGURE 18.2. Objective measurement of the effectiveness of the vacuum device for men with erectile dysfunction (*p < 0.01)

18.5 CONCLUSIONS FROM ORIGINAL REPORTS

These results confirm that the VD offers an effective, noninvasive therapy for erectile dysfunction. This study also demonstrates that the increase in penile volume resulting from the use of the VD was caused by arterial inflow as well as venous backflow, possibly because the vein valves do not function sufficiently under these unphysiological conditions.

18.6. STRENGTHS

The effects of the vacuum device were assessed both when it was used alone and when used in combination with a constriction ring. A variety of objective endpoints, e.g., Rigiscan and blood gas analysis, were employed, and nocturnal penile tumescence (NPT) was also evaluated.

18.7 WEAKNESSES

No attempt was made to determine a placebo response, e.g., by application of the device without application of the vacuum. All the conclusions are based on modest, generally non-statistically significant changes.

18.8 RELEVANCE

The parameters measured bear little relevance to the real-life use of such a device. However, the study does indicate that a vacuum device will offer an option for patients who do not want to use more invasive treatments or pharmacotherapy.

19. Study Descriptor
Pioneering Clinical Trial of Surgical Procedures

19.1 KEY TRIAL REFERENCES

19.1.1 Major Publication
Mulcahy J, Krane R, et al. Duraphase penile prosthesis – results of clinical trials in 63 patients. J Urol 143:518–519, 1990.

19.1.2 Other Important Publications
Govier F, Gibbons R, et al. Mechanical reliability, surgical complications, and patient and partner satisfaction of the modern three-piece inflatable penile prosthesis. Urology 52(2):282–286, 1998.

Sexton W, Benedict J, Jarrow J. Comparison of long-term outcomes of penile prostheses and intracavernosal injection therapy. J Urol 159(3):811–815, 1998.

19.2 IMPORTANCE OF STUDY
This was the first study in which the impact of a penile prosthetic was systematically followed up.

19.3 STUDY DESIGN
An open-label, multicenter, prospective study. n = 63.

A total of 63 patients were selected for implantation with the Duraphase prosthesis. Implantation of this semirigid rod prosthesis involves the placement of two cylinders, one in each of the corpora cavernosa. Each cylinder consists of a series of articulating segments (that give a good range of bendability) with a central steel cable attached to a spring at each end (to provide good axial rigidity).

The mean follow-up time for these patients was 4 months.

19.3.1 Outcome Measures
Treatment success was assessed by failure rate and patient satisfaction.

19.3.2 Inclusion Criteria

Men with erectile dysfunction (ED). The age range was 40 to 73 years (mean age, 59 years). The etiology of impotence was vasculogenic in 70%, diabetes in 27%, hypertension in 13%, neurological in 6%, drug-induced in 6%, and prostatectomy in 5%.

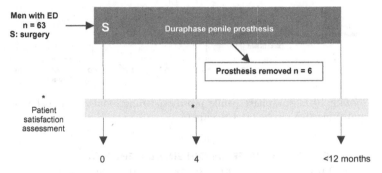

FIGURE 19.1. Duraphase penile prosthesis implantation: study design

19.4 KEY RESULTS

- In 6 patients, the prosthesis was removed within a year after implantation: 5 due to inadequate support and 1 because of intractable pain at 10 weeks.
- In 4 of the 5 patients in whom rigidity was insufficient, failure was due to cable fracture. In 2 of these patients, the Duraphase prosthesis was replaced, and the other 2 patients received an inflatable device. In the remaining patient (no cable failure), the problem of inadequate rigidity was improved by placement of the larger-gauge Duraphase prosthesis.
- Among the 57 patients in whom the original Duraphase prosthesis was still in place for at least 4 months, 55 patients were satisfied with the device. The reason for dissatisfaction was lack of sensitivity in 1 patient and an "unnatural" feeling in the other patient.
- Of these 57 patients, 52 had had satisfactory intercourse at 4 months.
- A good result was achieved in all 57 patients with respect to adequacy of support for intercourse and concealability during daily activities.

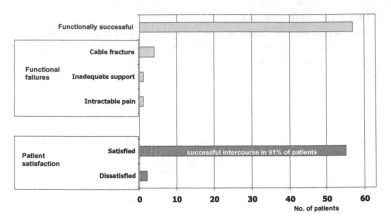

FIGURE 19.2. Duraphase penile prosthesis: functional results (<1 year) and subjective results (at 4 months)

19.5 CONCLUSIONS FROM ORIGINAL REPORTS

The Duraphase penile prosthesis proved a satisfactory treatment for ED in the majority of patients. The prosthesis was functionally successful in 90% of patients and was considered to be satisfactory by 87% of patients at 4 months following implantation.

The Duraphase prosthesis is easy to insert, has good axial rigidity, and is easy to bend and conceal, making it attractive to both physician and patient.

19.6 STRENGTHS

This is a quality publication covering the experience of four investigational sites in the USA.

19.7 WEAKNESSES

For obvious ethical reasons, a placebo could not be included. Assessment of patient and partner satisfaction used qualitative scoring systems only.

19.8 RELEVANCE

This study is likely to reflect the real-life success rate of good urological surgeons. In general, this particular device has been replaced by other variants.

Index